Emily Kerrigan

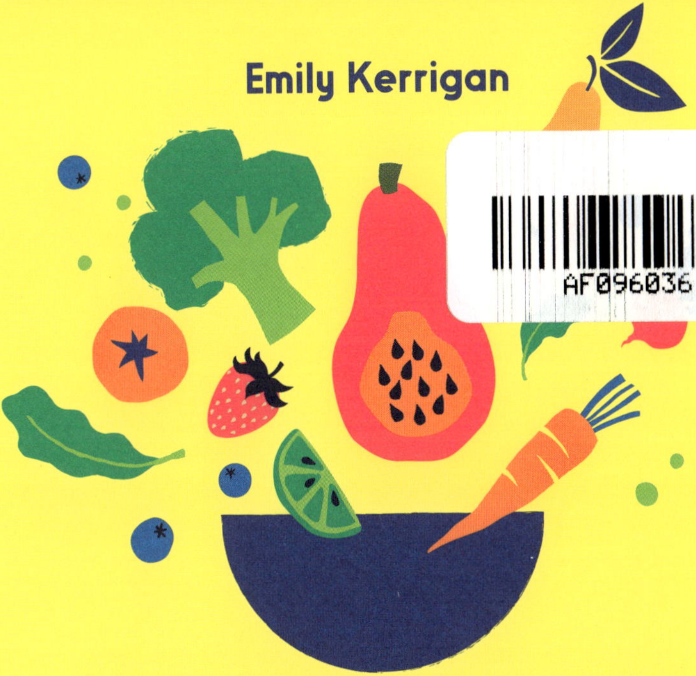

NUTRITION HACKS

Shortcuts and Healthy Swaps to Optimize Your Diet

vie

NUTRITION HACKS

Copyright © Octopus Publishing Group Limited, 2026

All rights reserved.

No part of this book may be reproduced by any means, nor transmitted, nor translated into a machine language, without the written permission of the publishers.

Emily Kerrigan has asserted their right to be identified as the author of this work in accordance with sections 77 and 78 of the Copyright, Designs and Patents Act 1988.

Condition of Sale
This book is sold subject to the condition that it shall not, by way of trade or otherwise, be lent, resold, hired out or otherwise circulated in any form of binding or cover other than that in which it is published and without a similar condition including this condition being imposed on the subsequent purchaser.

An Hachette UK Company
www.hachette.co.uk

Vie Books, an imprint of Summersdale Publishers
Part of Octopus Publishing Group Limited
Carmelite House
50 Victoria Embankment
LONDON
EC4Y 0DZ
UK

This FSC® label means that materials and other controlled sources used for the product have been responsibly sourced

www.summersdale.com

The authorized representative in the EEA is Hachette Ireland, 8 Castlecourt Centre, Dublin 15, D15 XTP3, Ireland (email: info@hbgi.ie)

Printed and bound in China

ISBN: 978-1-83799-741-1
eISBN: 978-1-83799-742-8

Substantial discounts on bulk quantities of Summersdale books are available to corporations, professional associations and other organizations. For details contact general enquiries: telephone: +44 (0) 1243 771107 or email: enquiries@summersdale.com.

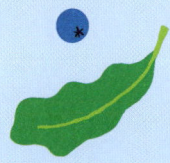

Contents

Introduction
5

Chapter One: Nutrition 101
7

Chapter Two: Food Myths
47

Chapter Three: Nutrition Hacks
64

Chapter Four: Weekly Meal Plans
151

Conclusion
158

Further Reading
159

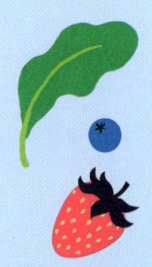

Disclaimer

Neither the author nor the publisher can be held responsible for any injury, loss or claim – be it health, financial or otherwise – arising out of the use, or misuse, of the suggestions made herein. Always consult your doctor before trying any new diet if you have a medical or health condition, or are worried about any of the side effects. This book is not intended as a substitute for the medical advice of a doctor or physician.

Introduction

If you've picked up this book, chances are you're thinking about making a few changes to your diet. What we choose to eat three times a day is a complicated thing, shaped by all kinds of factors from time and money to home life and community. Meanwhile, the noise around nutrition in retail and the media keeps getting louder, and misinformation is rife, making it increasingly tricky to distinguish fact from fiction.

This book cuts through all the confusion. It explains in simple, bite-sized entries exactly what good nutrition is and how you can best make it work for you. Along the way, we'll dispel a few myths so that you can choose foods based on scientific facts, not fads.

Which brings us to the hacks themselves: simple, fad-free, healthy habits we can all adopt to help us properly fuel our bodies. By the time we're done, you'll have all the tools you need, including delicious recipes for everyday eating and ready-made weekly meal plans. Either read the whole book from cover to cover or just dip in and out – you'll find page references throughout to help you join the dots between topics. Nutrition can be complex, but this little book is a simplified guide that can help every single one of us eat well every day.

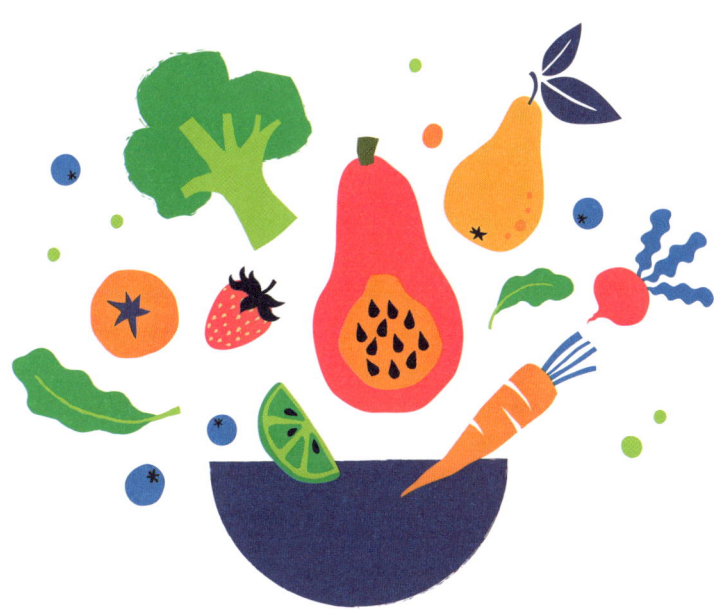

Chapter One:
NUTRITION 101

Before we start, let's get one thing straight: within a balanced diet, there is no such thing as "good" or "bad" food. Nutritious diets are about enjoying a variety of foods, and that can include both kale and cake. It's what we eat on repeat that matters for our health, not what we eat on occasion. This chapter covers everything you need to know about nutrition to help you make informed choices.

So what is a balanced diet?

The food you eat fuels your body. When you regularly feed your body the nutrients it needs, your physical health, mood, sleep quality, energy levels and ability to concentrate all benefit.

Foods can be made up of macronutrients (which are carbohydrates, protein and fat) and micronutrients (which are vitamins and minerals). We'll discuss all these separately in more detail over the coming pages. The three macronutrients provide the bulk of our nourishment, but micronutrients are no less vital – our body just requires them in tiny micro doses, hence the name.

The plate opposite illustrates the proportions of different foods we should aim to eat in a balanced diet. As a rule, try to make about 50% of your overall diet micronutrient-rich fruits and vegetables, 25% wholegrain carbohydrates and 25% lean protein and healthy fats. But don't think you need to stick to this rigidly; a balanced diet also means enjoying a celebratory meal out with friends or a guilt-free slice of birthday cake without overthinking it all. Just get back to eating in balance again the next day.

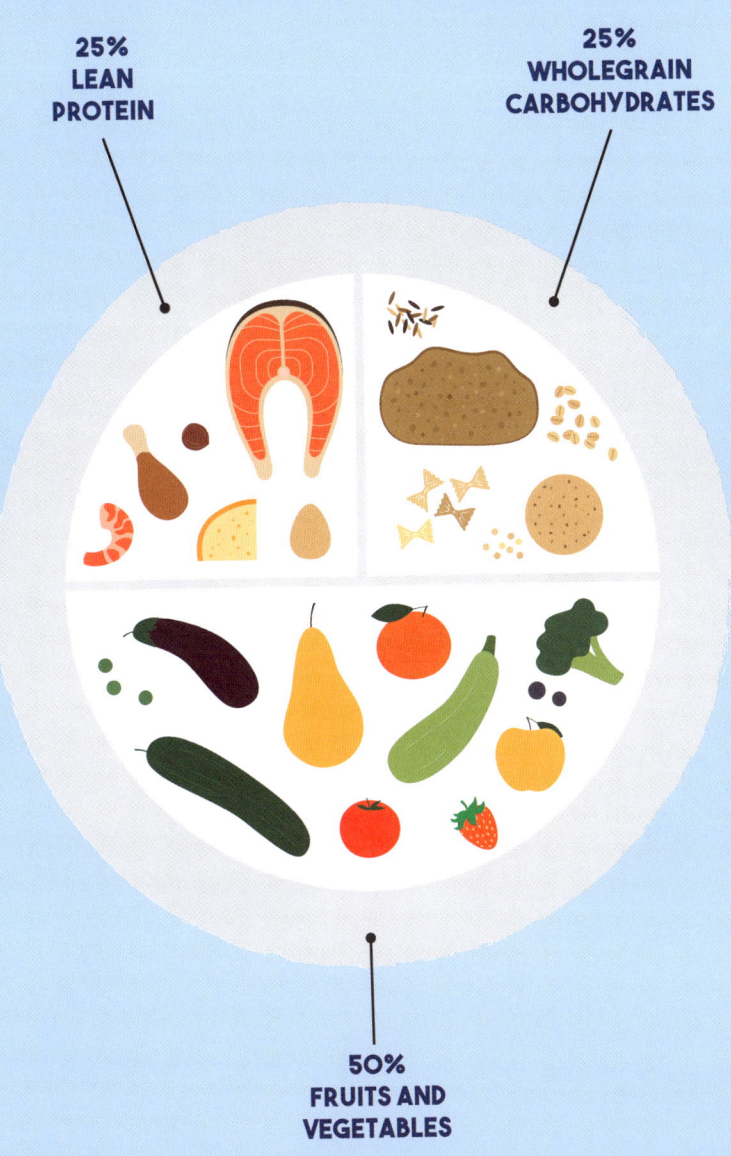

Carbohydrates

Most people think of carbs as starchy foods like white pasta or bread, but carbohydrates are in fruit, vegetables and legumes, too. Carbohydrates are our body and brain's main source of energy. All carbs provide glucose, which we either use immediately or convert into glycogen and store to use later (read more on p.56). But some carbs are more useful than others.

The picture opposite shows examples of high- and low-quality carbohydrates. High-quality carbohydrates are excellent natural sources of vitamins, minerals and fibre. By contrast, low-quality carbs are refined, often high in sugar and/or saturated fat or salt and have had any fibre removed during processing. Fibre is good for our gut, and fibre-rich, complex carbohydrates are a stable source of energy because they take longer to digest.

You can make simple swaps every day to improve the quality of carbs you eat: instead of sugary breakfast cereal, switch to porridge or overnight oats; in place of a white bagel at lunch, use brown or seeded bread; and rather than white rice with dinner, cook different wholegrains, like quinoa or brown rice.

HIGH-QUALITY CARBOHYDRATES

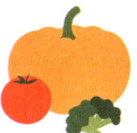

vegetables

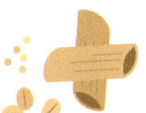

wholegrains

fruit

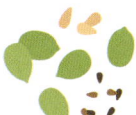

seeds

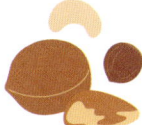

nuts

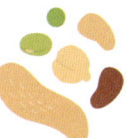

beans

LOW-QUALITY CARBOHYDRATES

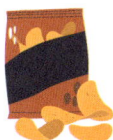

crisps

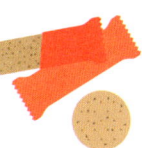

biscuits

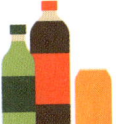

sugary drinks

sweets

fast food

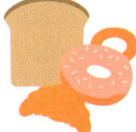

bakery items

Carbohydrates and blood sugar

Carbohydrates consist of either simple or complex sugars. Examples of simple carbohydrates are refined white flour, fruit, honey and dairy; complex carbs are vegetables, pulses and unrefined wholegrains. All carbohydrates raise blood sugar, but glucose from simple carbs is released into our bloodstream at speed, whilst complex carbs take longer to break down and release glucose.

The Glycaemic Index (GI) measures how quickly foods raise blood glucose. High-GI foods cause rapid spikes, whereas low-GI foods provide more stable energy by releasing glucose slowly. The odd spike from a slice of cake isn't normally anything to fret over (see p.49), but it's best to eat mainly complex carbs, as doing so avoids fluctuations in blood sugar which can cause tiredness, hunger and mood swings.

The GI can be a useful guide but it isn't a perfect measure. There's no need to get too concerned about the numbers, and some of them are even misleading. A slice of watermelon is a high-GI simple carb, for example, as is a cookie (see opposite), but watermelon is a healthy snack and one of your five a day. It scores high on the Index because it contains fruit sugar – but it also provides fibre and vitamins, making it an excellent choice for a snack and significantly more nutrient-dense than a cookie.

TOP TIPS

Aim to eat mostly complex carbs, and "dress up" your carbs by eating them alongside protein and healthy fats. This further helps slow down carb absorption and curbs sugar spikes.

GLYCAEMIC INDEX

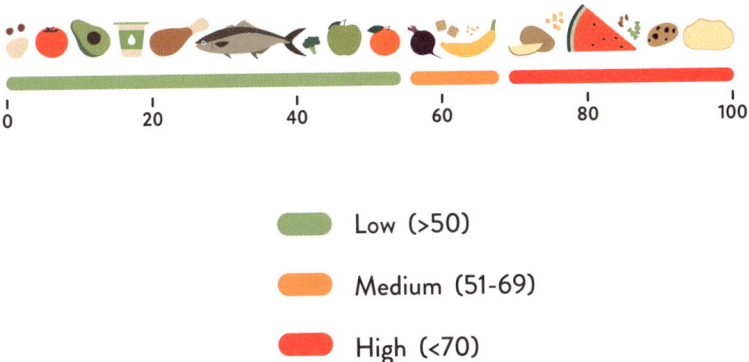

- Low (>50)
- Medium (51-69)
- High (<70)

Carbohydrates and fibre

Fibre is part of a complex carbohydrate that we cannot break down and use for fuel. But fibre has many uses all the same. As it passes slowly undigested through the gut, it keeps us feeling fuller for longer, which reduces the likelihood of weight gain. It keeps blood sugars stable by slowing down glucose absorption, plus it lowers cholesterol – this is especially true of a type of fibre called "beta glucan" found in oats and barley. Together, these reduce the risk of heart disease and type 2 diabetes.

Fibre also keeps us regular. There are two types, soluble and insoluble, often found in the same foods. Soluble fibre is in the flesh of fruit and veg, plus wholegrains, legumes and pulses. It absorbs water in the gut, softening stools. Insoluble is in the skin and seeds of fruit and veg, as well as wholegrains, nuts and seeds. It adds bulk, helping stools pass through the gut.

Most of us don't eat enough fibre. We should aim for 30 g a day but the average intake is more like 18 g. Find hacks for meeting your target on p.72, more about gut health on p.32, plus recipes with fibre-rich pulses and beans on p.124.

SOLUBLE FIBRE

vegetables

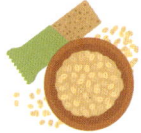
oats

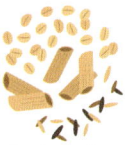
wholegrains

fruit

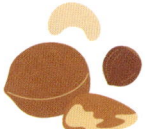
nuts

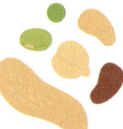
beans

INSOLUBLE FIBRE

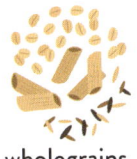
wholegrains

fruit

vegetables

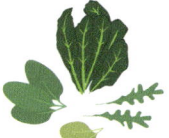
greens

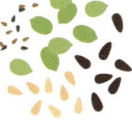
seeds

sprouts

Protein

Our bodies contain thousands of different proteins – think of them as our building blocks. We need protein to form and repair everything from tissues, muscles and skin to hair and nails. All proteins consist of amino acids, and there are 20 specific amino acids we need to function. We can make all but nine within the body – these nine are the essential amino acids and we must get them from food. We can't store protein like we can carbohydrates and fat, so we need to consume it every day.

Animal products (dairy, eggs, fish and meat) are known as "complete" proteins because they contain all nine essential amino acids. So do a few plant sources, like soya, quinoa, chia seeds and buckwheat. If you don't eat any animal products, you can instead combine "incomplete" plant proteins to get all nine on one plate. This isn't as complicated as it sounds; baked beans on wholegrain toast is a straightforward example of protein combining, as is combining black beans with brown rice, pasta with peas, or oats with nuts.

ANIMAL PROTEIN

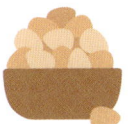
eggs

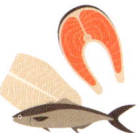
fish

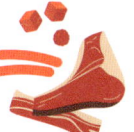
meat

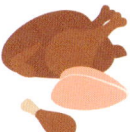
poultry

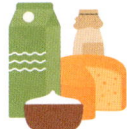
dairy

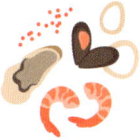
seafood

PLANT PROTEIN

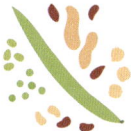
legumes

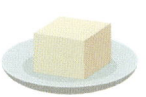
tofu

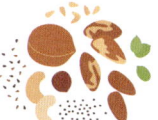
nuts and seeds

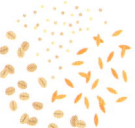
wholegrains

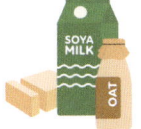
plant-based fortified foods

vegetables

Protein and portions

Try to include a portion of protein in every meal. It keeps you feeling fuller for longer and slows absorption of the carbs you eat with it. On average, we should aim to eat about 0.75 g of protein per kg of body weight per day. If you're very active, eating some extra protein within an hour of hard exercise will help your body recover and repair muscle.

Simple variations for adding more protein to breakfast include porridge or Greek yoghurt topped with seeds, wholemeal toast spread with nut butters, or eggs. At lunch and dinner, opt for lean chicken, seafood, fish or tofu and include plenty of beans, grains, lentils and pulses. For an easy protein snack, spread an oatcake with houmous or apple slices with nut butter.

If you eat animal protein, focus on lean poultry, eggs or dairy and less on red meat. Limit processed meat. Include two portions of fish a week, one of which is oily. For more on plant-based protein, see p.30.

TOP TIPS

It's always best to get protein from nutrient-dense real food first. Most people can get more than enough from the foods they eat without the need for extra supplements (see more on p.61).

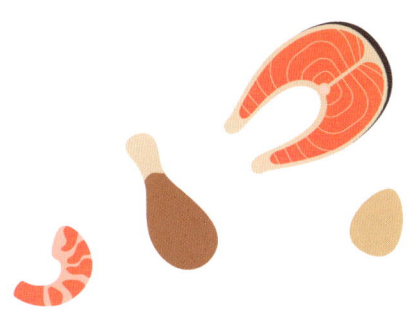

Types of fat

Fat sometimes suffers with an image problem, but not all fat is bad. Fat is vital for our wellbeing, giving us energy, helping us feel full and adding flavour to food. We need healthy fats to support cell and hormone production, as well as brain function. Moreover, there is a group of vitamins that our body cannot absorb without some fat in our diet (these are known as the fat-soluble vitamins A, D, E and K).

All fat is higher in energy than the other two macronutrients: one gram of fat provides nine calories, whereas one gram of either carbohydrate or protein provides four calories. Excess fat that isn't used in our cells, or for fuel, gets converted into body fat. To maintain a healthy weight, we therefore need to be mindful of how much we eat.

The picture opposite illustrates sources of saturated and unsaturated fat. To reduce the risk of heart disease, we should opt mainly for unsaturated fat and only eat saturated fat in moderation.

SATURATED FAT

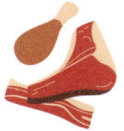
fatty meat

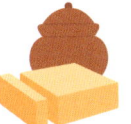
butter

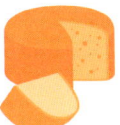
cheese

milk, cream

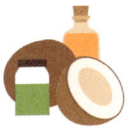
coconut oil

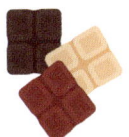
chocolate

UNSATURATED FAT

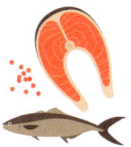
fatty fish

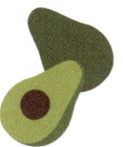
avocado

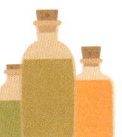
plant oils

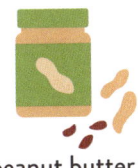
peanut butter

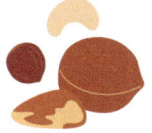
nuts

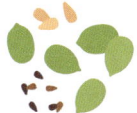
seeds

Healthy fats

Healthy unsaturated fats can be monounsaturated or polyunsaturated. Both help lower "bad" low-density lipoprotein (LDL) cholesterol (read more on p.58) in our blood and support heart health. Sources of monounsaturated fat include olive and rapeseed oils, avocados, Brazil nuts and peanuts.

There are two main types of polyunsaturated fats: omega-3 and omega-6. Most of us get enough omega-6, which is in vegetable oils and nuts. Ensure you get enough omega-3, though, which is only found in less commonly eaten foods, like oily fish. Aim for two portions of fish a week, one of them oily fish, like salmon, mackerel or trout. Plant-based sources of omega-3 include chia, hemp and flaxseeds.

Overall, we should get about a third of our calories from healthy fats, but not more – that's about 70 g of fat a day. To give you an idea of what that looks like, half an avocado provides about 12 g, 1 tablespoon of nut butter about 7 g, and a steamed skinless salmon fillet about 19 g.

Dairy

Dairy is an excellent source of protein, calcium, iodine, phosphorus, potassium and B vitamins. Some fermented dairy foods, like live yoghurt or kefir, also contain gut-friendly probiotics (learn more on p.33).

All the same, dairy can be high in saturated fat and should be eaten in moderation (think of creamy sauces, butter or cheese). Opt instead for lower-fat versions for day-to-day use, such as semi-skimmed or skimmed milk, cottage cheese or lower-fat cream cheese. Remember that all products labelled "lower fat" still contain some fat. Moreover, some low-fat alternatives, such as yoghurts, are not necessarily lower in calories because the fat may have been replaced with additional sugar. Always check labels so that you know what you're buying. Unsweetened, reduced-fat Greek or natural live yoghurt is the most nutritious bet.

If you're vegan, ensure you include unsweetened plant-based dairy alternatives that are fortified with calcium, iodine and B vitamins.

Vitamins

We need vitamins in small but vital doses to keep us healthy and our body functioning at its best. The picture opposite illustrates some food sources of each.

- Vitamin A (or retinol) boosts immunity, keeps skin healthy and is essential for vision. Yellow and orange fruits and vegetables contain beta-carotene, a natural pigment that can be converted to retinol in the body. Retinol itself is found in meat, dairy, eggs and oily fish.

- B vitamins help release energy from food and support our nervous system. Vitamin B6 (pyridoxine) also helps make haemoglobin, the substance in red blood cells that transports oxygen.

- Vitamin B9 (folate) supports foetal brain and spinal cord development during pregnancy; a lack may also cause anaemia.

- Vitamin B12 (cobalamin) helps make red blood cells. It's found in meat, fish and dairy, so vegans are advised to supplement and eat fortified plant foods.

- Vitamin C is a powerful antioxidant that protects cells, aids wound healing and maintains healthy skin, blood vessels and cartilage.

- We get vitamin D, needed for healthy bones, from sunlight, as well as egg yolks, oily fish, red meat, mushrooms and fortified foods. During the shorter days of winter, we should all supplement; pregnant and breastfeeding women, children under 5, adults over 65, and those who get little sun exposure or have darker skin should supplement year-round.
- Vitamin E supports immunity, alongside healthy skin and eyes.
- Vitamin K is needed for blood clotting and wound healing. Studies indicate it may also keep bones healthy.

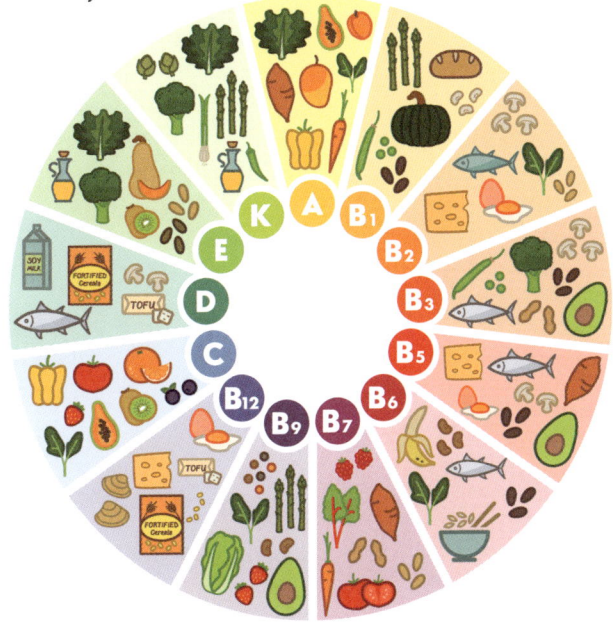

Minerals

Just like vitamins, we need minerals in micro doses to keep us healthy. The following pictures show some example food sources of each mineral and why we need them.

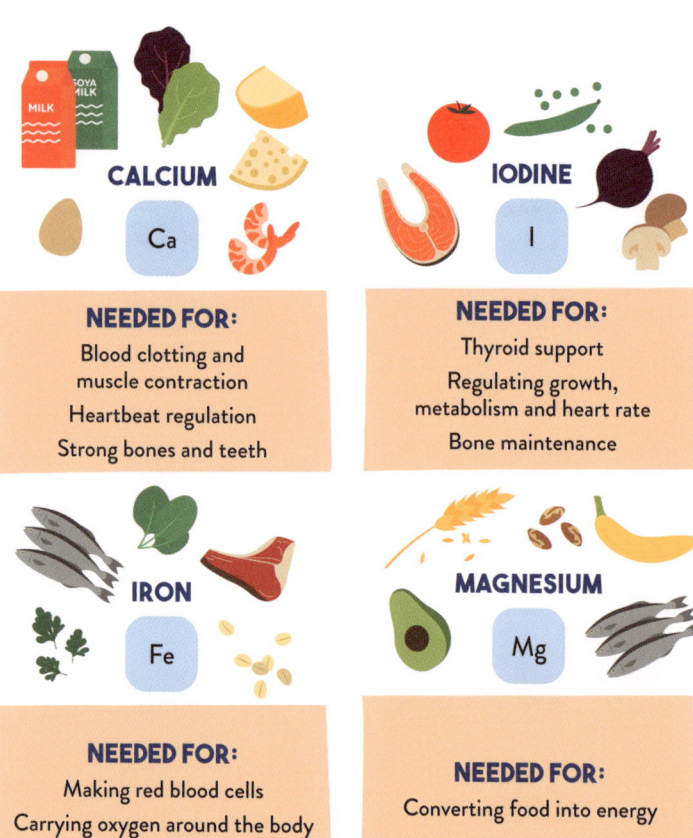

CALCIUM

Ca

NEEDED FOR:

Blood clotting and muscle contraction

Heartbeat regulation

Strong bones and teeth

IODINE

I

NEEDED FOR:

Thyroid support

Regulating growth, metabolism and heart rate

Bone maintenance

IRON

Fe

NEEDED FOR:

Making red blood cells

Carrying oxygen around the body

MAGNESIUM

Mg

NEEDED FOR:

Converting food into energy

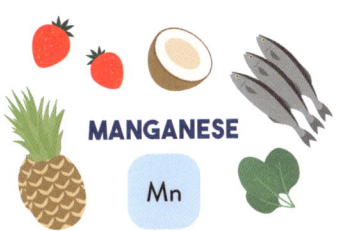

MANGANESE
Mn

NEEDED FOR:
Chemical reactions including breaking down food

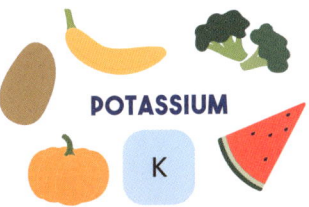

POTASSIUM
K

NEEDED FOR:
Controlling fluid balance

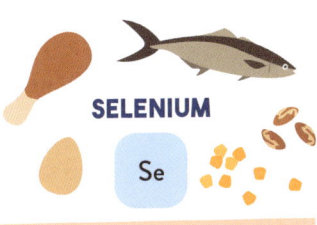

SELENIUM
Se

NEEDED FOR:
Supporting our immune and reproductive systems

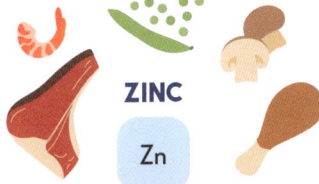

ZINC
Zn

NEEDED FOR:
Wound healing

Eating the rainbow

The best way to get all the vitamins and minerals you need is to eat a balanced diet, including a rainbow of micronutrient-rich fruits and vegetables. Colourful and delicious, fruit and veg are also high in fibre and polyphenols – powerful plant chemicals containing antioxidants which protect our cells from damage. Different coloured plants provide different polyphenols – for example, red fruits like tomatoes contain one called lycopene, whilst purple fruit and veg are rich in another called an anthocyanin.

Eating five portions a day of fruit and veg lowers the risk of heart disease, stroke and some cancers. What counts towards your five a day? One portion is 80 g of fresh, canned or frozen fruit or veg (80 g is about the size of your clenched fist). If it's canned, choose tins with no added sugar or salt.

You can also count a portion of fibre-rich beans or pulses as one of your five a day (even though they're not fruit or veg). Potatoes don't count unless they're sweet potatoes. Standard potatoes are still nutritious, though: potato salads contain gut-loving resistant starch (see p.32), whilst baked potatoes are full of fibre, especially if you eat the skin and pile them high with salad.

TOP TIPS

To benefit both general and gut health, aim to eat 30 plants a week: these include fruit, veg, beans, pulses, legumes, nuts, seeds, grains, herbs and spices. You'll find simple ways to add more plants to your diet on pp.70–71.

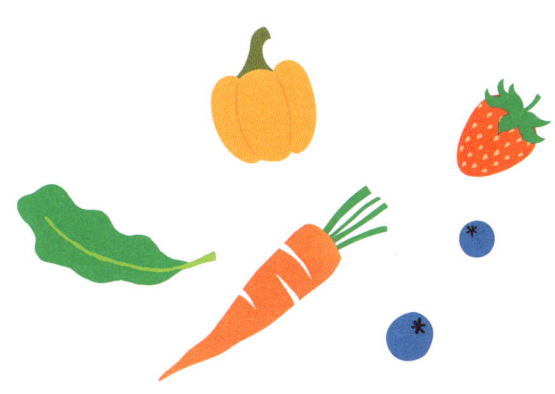

Plant-based diets

The term "plant-based" means different things to different people; flexitarians and some omnivores might base their diets predominantly on plants, for example, whereas vegans base it exclusively so. A well-planned plant-based diet can be hugely beneficial for the planet as well as your health – but only if you ensure you get all the nutrients you need and don't rely on ultra-processed plant-based foods.

For vegetarians who eat dairy and eggs, a balanced diet is as described from p.8, minus meat and fish. Pulses, tofu, tempeh, edamame and quinoa are examples of quality plant protein to replace meat and fish, and protein combining is important (see p.16). Ensure ample iron (from pulses, dried apricots, dark green veg, nuts, fortified cereals and wholemeal bread), as well as vitamin B12 (from milk, cheese, eggs, plus yeast extract and nutritional yeast, fortified cereals and fortified soya products). In place of omega-3s found in oily fish, vegetarians should eat plenty of flaxseed and rapeseed oils, chia and hemp seeds, walnuts and eggs enriched with omega-3.

Those eating a vegan diet should follow the above advice regarding protein and iron. Vegan sources of omega-3 are as above, minus the fish and eggs. Plant sources of calcium are calcium-set tofu, fortified unsweetened plant milks, tahini, pulses, dried apricots and green leafy veg (excluding spinach, which inhibits calcium absorption).

Vegans should supplement with vitamin D, vitamin B12, iodine, selenium, calcium and iron – or ensure they get enough from fortified foods and plant sources.

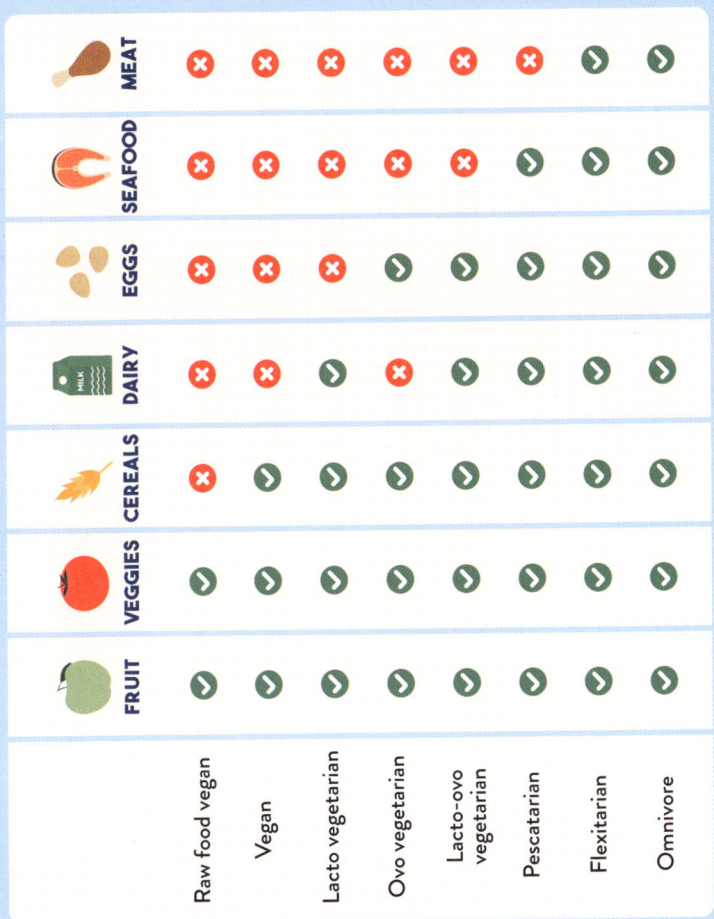

	Raw food vegan	Vegan	Lacto vegetarian	Ovo vegetarian	Lacto-ovo vegetarian	Pescatarian	Flexitarian	Omnivore
MEAT	✗	✗	✗	✗	✗	✗	✓	✓
SEAFOOD	✗	✗	✗	✗	✗	✓	✓	✓
EGGS	✗	✗	✗	✓	✓	✓	✓	✓
DAIRY	✗	✗	✓	✗	✓	✓	✓	✓
CEREALS	✗	✓	✓	✓	✓	✓	✓	✓
VEGGIES	✓	✓	✓	✓	✓	✓	✓	✓
FRUIT	✓	✓	✓	✓	✓	✓	✓	✓

Food for a happy gut

Eating plant-based meals – wherever you sit on the scale on p.31 – keeps your gut healthy. We all play host to trillions of good bacteria within our gut microbiome. These friendly bugs help digestion and boost immunity and general wellbeing. Moreover, there's growing evidence linking gut health to mood (this pathway is called the gut–brain axis). The more diverse and numerous our good gut bacteria, the better. And the more diverse and numerous the plants we eat, the more these good bacteria thrive.

Friendly gut bacteria feed off plant polyphenols and fibre, turning them into valuable nutrients called short-chain fatty acids (SCFAs). Starchy carbs like rice, potatoes and pasta also help form these SCFAs. If you cook potatoes, rice or pasta, then allow them to cool down, they form something called resistant starch. This is fermented during digestion to produce SCFAs, which feed the gut lining.

Meanwhile, a diet low in plants and high in saturated fat, salt and sugar can imbalance our gut microbiome, causing an overgrowth of less beneficial bacteria. Stress, antibiotics and lack of exercise or sleep also imbalance gut bacteria.

Pre- and probiotic supplements are marketed as beneficial for maintaining gut balance. Research suggests they're helpful to restore your microbiome following antibiotics.

Some foods are naturally prebiotic, meaning they boost existing friendly bacteria. These include apples, leeks, onions, garlic, artichokes and asparagus. Probiotic foods, meanwhile, deliver all-new friendly bacteria to the gut. Fermented foods like live yoghurt, pickles, kimchi and miso are all probiotics.

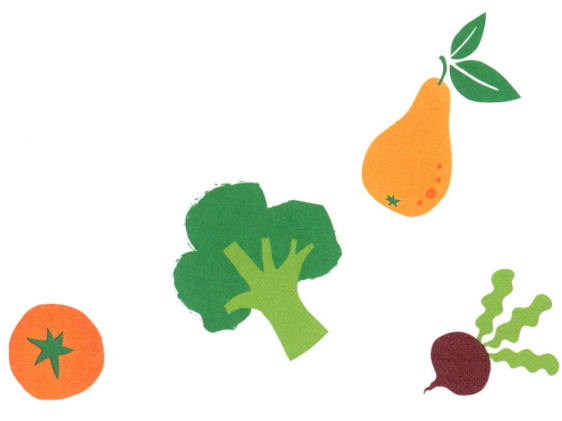

Understanding food labels

Whether you're buying groceries to cook with or choosing a snack on the go, reading the packaging can help you make informed choices about the foods you buy.

Some packaging includes traffic-light labelling – an at-a-glance indication of a food's saturated fat, sugar and salt content. Choose mostly foods lower in these and labelled green (and/or amber for medium). Limit those labelled red which indicates they're high in fat, sugar or salt.

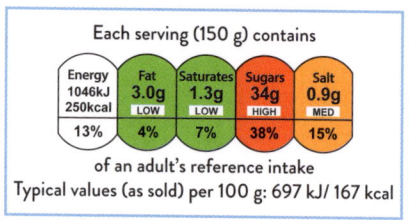

OHID in association with the Welsh government, Food Standards Scotland and the Food Standards Agency in Northern Ireland.

All 14 food allergens must also be declared on packaging. If you think you may have a food allergy or intolerance, always speak to a health professional to get correctly diagnosed. Keep a food diary to monitor symptoms and triggers. The 14 most common allergens are celery, gluten, crustaceans, eggs, fish, lupin flour, milk, molluscs, mustard, peanuts, sesame, soybeans, tree nuts, and sulphur dioxide and sulphites.

HFSS foods

Most of us eat too many HFSS (high in fat, sugar and salt) foods.

Women should eat less than 20 g a day of saturated fat and men less than 30 g. Too much can raise cholesterol (see p.58) and risk heart disease. Foods high in saturated fat include fatty cuts of meat, butter and cream.

Free sugars can cause weight gain and tooth decay. A free sugar is any that is added to food and drink, plus the sugar in fruit juice, honey and syrups. Adults should eat no more than 30 g a day (a regular can of Coke contains 35 g). Free sugars hide in savoury processed foods, too, like soups or salad dressings, and go by many names including sucrose, dextrose, brown rice syrup and corn syrup.

Too much salt puts us at risk of high blood pressure and heart disease. Adults should eat less than 6 g a day (about one teaspoon). Salt is common in processed foods including ketchup, soy sauce, pastries, cheese and processed meats. Some pizzas can contain as much as 14 g!

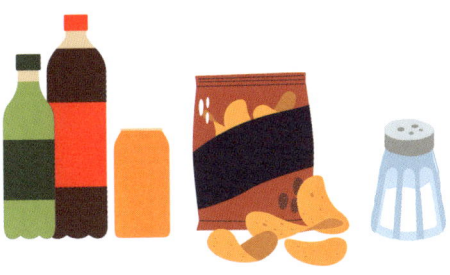

Ultra-processed and fast foods

Foods are classified according to the degree of processing they've been through. Not all processed food is unhealthy (see more on p.50) but often these processes can impact a food's nutritional value, as this example of fat and salt content in different potato products illustrates:

POTATO VERSUS PROCESSING

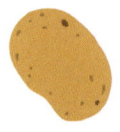 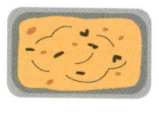 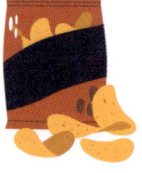 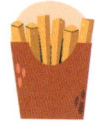

UNPROCESSED **PROCESSED** **UPF** **FAST FOOD**

fat fat fat fat

salt salt salt salt

Ultra-processed foods (UPFs) and fast foods are hard to avoid: they're manufactured to be extremely palatable, accessible, convenient and affordable. But a diet high in these foods isn't good for us for two reasons. Firstly, UPFs and fast foods tend to be both calorific and HFSS foods, increasing our risk of obesity, type 2 diabetes and heart disease. Secondly, they're mostly low in the nutrients we need, like wholegrains, fibre, lean protein, fruits and vegetables.

The hacks in this book can help if you'd like to reduce UPFs and fast foods in favour of a more balanced diet based on fresh foods. Fresh foods can be accessible, convenient and affordable, too, not to mention delicious.

Food for a healthy body

Eating a balanced diet helps keep you feeling your best. It boosts gut health and immunity, improves sleep, bolsters energy levels, supports concentration and helps us maintain a healthy weight.

A poor diet centred around HFSS foods and lacking wholegrains, fruits and vegetables does the reverse. Poor diets are associated with heart disease and weight gain – and obesity increases the risk of cancer and type 2 diabetes.

Healthy eating needn't be complicated. Start by introducing new little habits that in time become fixed, leading to long-term health gains. But avoid guilt and the unrealistic expectation that your diet needs to be perfect.

The decisions we make about the foods we eat are shaped by practical considerations like time, affordability and accessibility. Meals often involve shortcuts and compromises. Eating well for health is about the bigger picture. Food is for enjoyment, too, and not just fuel. Eating all kinds of foods in balance, including the odd less nutrient-dense one, is part of that bigger picture, too.

Food for a healthy weight

Many people approach healthy eating as a vehicle for losing weight. Restrictive weight-loss diets tend to be a short-term fix as they're hard to sustain. It can be more effective to find a way of healthy eating that works for you in the long term; you're more likely to stick to a balanced approach and lose weight steadily. Rather than excluding foods, focus instead on what to include: wholegrains, fruits, vegetables, alongside healthier versions of dishes you enjoy.

Men should consume 2,500 calories a day and women 2,000. Calorie counting is time-consuming, however, and doesn't offer the full picture because foods provide nutrients and not just energy. If you use a fitness tracker, it'll only be as accurate as the data you input, and we often underestimate the portions we eat. Whilst some people find it helpful to calorie count or step on the scales, for others it can become compulsive. Do seek professional support if you feel you have an unhealthy relationship with food or have any concerns about your weight.

Food for a healthy mind

To help us concentrate, our brain needs sufficient energy; in fact, our brain uses one fifth of all our body's energy needs. Our brain gets energy from blood glucose derived from the carbohydrates we eat. When we eat high-quality carbohydrates, our brain benefits from a steady supply of fuel; eating low-quality carbs results instead in spikes and crashes to blood glucose. These rollercoasters are associated with poor concentration and mood swings. It's not surprising, then, that a Mediterranean diet (see p.44), which centres on high-quality carbs like wholegrains and vegetables, has been linked in some studies to improved mood. Omega-3s (such as oily fish, walnuts and chia seeds) also support the brain.

Additionally, researchers are interested in the gut–brain axis and how our gut microbiome might impact the way we feel. Others are investigating serotonin, a chemical messenger in our brain which improves mood. Serotonin is made from an amino acid called tryptophan, so it may be that eating protein foods containing tryptophan (like chicken, milk, eggs and soybeans) boosts mood, too.

Mindful and intuitive eating

Mindful and intuitive eating can realign our mindset around food. Mindful eating is taking the time to enjoy food without distractions – when we eat a snack whilst scrolling through our phone without really registering it, we're eating mindlessly. With mindful eating we remove distractions, slow down and relish our food, meaning we're more likely to choose suitable portions and recognize when we're full.

Intuitive eating encourages us to ditch dieting and avoid food restriction. Instead, we should enjoy a balanced diet, eating when hungry and stopping when full. Intuitive eating centres on positive body image. Exercise is encouraged for enjoyment, not to burn calories or "permit" the eating of certain foods.

These two approaches may not be suitable if you or someone you know might be suffering with disordered eating. Eating disorders do not discriminate and can affect anyone, but studies tell us that recovery is possible at any time. If you need support, do ensure you get specialist help (resources on p.159).

Hunger and hormones

Our bodies experience different types of hunger, controlled by different hormones. Homeostatic hunger means needing to eat for energy – it's the hunger we register when we feel tired, or our stomach growls. When our stomach is empty we release the hunger hormone ghrelin and when we are full, we release leptin. Together these guide our appetite.

Hedonic hunger is eating for pleasure. When we eat something delicious, our brain releases dopamine, a pleasure hormone. We then associate that food with feelings of pleasure, meaning we desire it even if we aren't hungry. Hedonic hunger explains why we might feel hungry when we see fast food advertising or pick up a tub of popcorn before watching a movie, regardless of whether or not we feel homeostatic hunger in that moment.

If you regularly experience hedonic hunger, it can help to eat foods that are high in fibre or protein, both of which increase satiation (feeling satisfied).

Exercise and sleep

Exercise boosts energy, self-esteem and mood and is an excellent stress buster. It lowers the risk of heart disease, type 2 diabetes and cancer whilst helping us maintain a healthy weight.

We should all move our bodies every day, aiming for 150 minutes of moderate activity a week, plus muscle strengthening twice weekly. This needn't necessarily be at the gym; brisk walking, taking the stairs instead of the lift and carrying heavy groceries count, too, just like swimming or sit-ups. Find leisure activities you enjoy and set yourself targets, perhaps committing to a challenge with others or enrolling in a team sport.

Regular exercise alongside good nutrition also helps us sleep well. By contrast, poor sleep disrupts hormones, increasing ghrelin and decreasing leptin (see opposite). This leads to snacking, overeating and potential weight gain over time. Getting enough sleep also helps control cortisol, the body's stress hormone.

Eating well for longevity

Modern diets have moved towards too many HFSS foods and away from wholegrains, fruits and vegetables. These diets are associated with an increased risk of heart disease, obesity and type 2 diabetes.

But in some parts of the world, more traditional diets still prevail. Nutritionists highlight three traditional eating patterns in particular – the Mediterranean, Nordic and Japanese diets – all of which share many elements of the balanced diet described in this chapter. According to research, in these countries people live longer, healthier and happier lives. It follows, then, that if we can incorporate more of these elements into our own meals and follow a similarly balanced (and delicious!) diet, then we can live longer, healthier and happier lives, too.

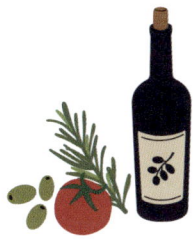
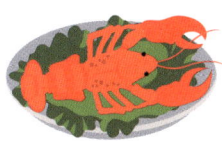
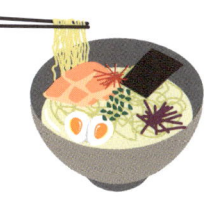

MEDITERRANEAN
fruit, vegetables, pulses, wholegrains, nuts and seeds

oily fish, lean poultry, yoghurt, cheese, eggs, olive oil

NORDIC
fruit, especially berries, legumes and wholegrains

oily fish, shellfish, low-fat dairy, eggs, rapeseed oil

JAPANESE
shiitake, rice, radishes, seaweed, ginger, matcha and sesame

oily fish, soybeans and soya, foods including tofu and miso

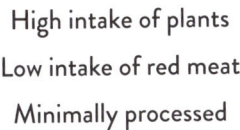

High intake of plants

Low intake of red meat

Minimally processed

The future of food

The decisions we make about our food can have a powerful impact on our own health and the health of the planet. Across the globe, administrations are wrestling to reduce the twin burdens of climate change and preventable illnesses such as heart disease and type 2 diabetes. Almost two thirds of deaths worldwide from preventable illnesses relate to poor diet, physical inactivity, harmful drinking or tobacco. Meanwhile, food systems are responsible for one third of human-generated carbon emissions.

Combined with regular exercise, eating a sustainable and balanced diet can make everyone's future look different. Switching to fresh ingredients in place of pre-prepared food as well as cutting down on red meat can have huge benefits for both your health and the planet.

Lastly, only take advice from registered nutritionists (see p.159), remembering that the headlines or products promoted by others may be manufactured around half-truths. The next chapter dispels some common myths you don't need to buy into.

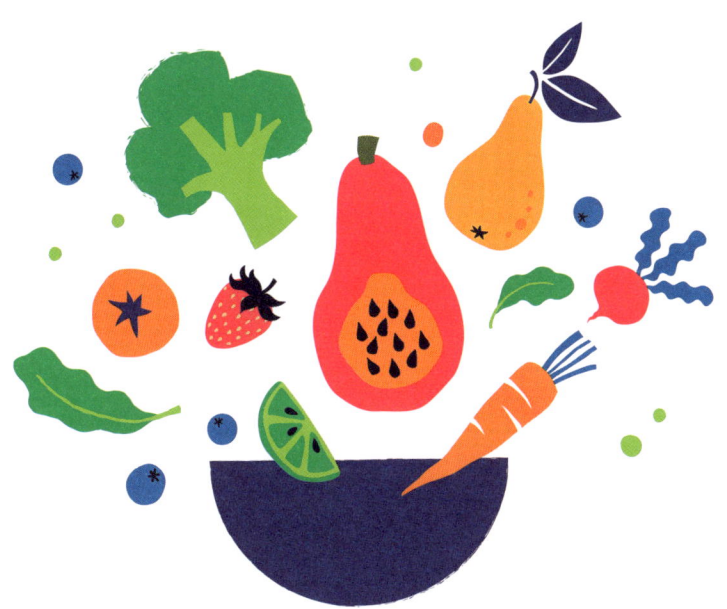

Chapter Two:
FOOD MYTHS

The internet is rife with misinformation about nutrition, often peddled by people trying to sell you something, from a fad diet to a clickbait headline. Advice from registered nutritionists and healthcare providers is valid and science-based. Take anything else with a pinch of salt and ask yourself if the person offering the advice is qualified to do so. This chapter dispels common myths you may have been mis-sold.

Myth 1: Fad diets are the key to weight loss

Research tells us that fad weight-loss diets don't work in the long term and that most people regain any weight they have lost within a year. It also indicates that no single weight-loss programme is any more effective than another, be that a low-fat, low-carb or high-protein diet.

Rather than following the latest craze, counting calories, skipping meals, limiting certain foods or yo-yo dieting, it is more effective to find a sustainable overall approach to healthy eating that works for you. Eating a balanced diet and losing weight slowly and steadily has been proven to be the most effective way. Listen to your body, eating when you're hungry and stopping when you're full. Enjoy healthy snacks and keep an eye on portions. Don't deprive yourself of less healthy foods that you like – just eat them in moderation. Get enough exercise and sleep, be kind to yourself and remember that food is for nourishment and enjoyment, not just fuel.

Myth 2: Sugar spikes need monitoring

Continuous glucose monitors (CGMs) were once reserved for patients with diabetes, but are now widely available from biotech companies marketing the idea that such personalized nutritional data is worthwhile. All the same, it's only people with diabetes who need monitors. When we eat, our blood sugar rises and our body produces insulin in response to regulate it. People with diabetes either cannot make, or have problems using, insulin and must monitor their glucose.

Some foods have a high Glycaemic Index that can spike blood sugar, but the odd spike after a cookie isn't normally anything to worry about if your sugars are balanced most of the time. Eating fibre-rich complex carbohydrates and pairing them with protein and healthy fats helps keep blood sugar balanced. Personalized nutrition is an emerging – and very lucrative – field of nutrition and it's up to you if you want to try a CGM. But if you're healthy, there's no need to get bogged down in it all and to do so risks stripping enjoyment out of eating.

Myth 3: All processed foods are unhealthy

We benefit from processed foods every day and it's both unrealistic and unnecessary to try to eliminate them. Some processing keeps us safe, like pasteurizing milk. Other processing gives us access to convenient, affordable, nutrient-dense food year-round, like frozen fruits and vegetables, canned fish or bottles of olive oil. The NOVA scale (pictured opposite) categorizes food processing into levels. We should aim to eat mostly group 1 and 2 foods, keeping an eye on the saturated fat, salt and sugar we consume in group 2 and 3 foods and limiting ultra-processed foods. Processed ready meals are often expensive and high in salt, sugar and saturated fat, so limit your consumption of these by cooking meals from scratch at home instead. You'll simultaneously increase your intake of nutrient-dense foods, like wholegrains and vegetables, and, if you batch-cook and budget, you'll save time and money, too.

GROUP ONE
Unprocessed or minimally processed foods

Fresh, dry or frozen fruit and vegetables; grains; legumes; meat; fish; eggs; nuts; seeds

GROUP TWO
Processed culinary ingredients

Plant oils and animal fats; maple syrup; sugar; honey; salt

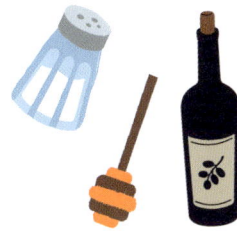

GROUP THREE
Processed foods

Canned/pickled vegetables, fruit, meat and fish; bread; cheese; salted meats; wine; beer; cider

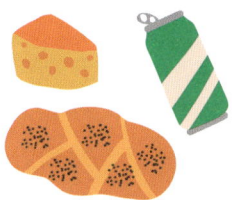

GROUP FOUR
Ultra-processed foods

Sugary beverages; packaged snacks; reconstituted meat products (e.g. sausages, ham, nuggets); ready meals; canned/instant soups; ice cream

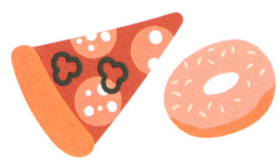

Myth 4: Plant-based diets are always nutritious

Choosing to follow a vegan or vegetarian diet is only as healthy as the day-to-day food choices you make within either eating pattern. Plant-based diets can offer excellent nutrition and lower our risk of disease but only if they are well-planned and balanced. If you cut out animal products and fish from your diet, you may lack protein, calcium, iron, vitamin B12, iodine, selenium and omega-3. Vegetarians can find many of these nutrients in eggs or dairy but vegans should look to fortified foods (see p.31). In particular, be aware that many plant-based ultra-processed foods can be high in saturated fat, salt and sugar. If the majority of your plant-based diet consists of these rather than fresh fruit and vegetables, wholegrains, quality plant protein and healthy fats, then it won't be nutritious at all.

Myth 5: Your gut needs a cleanse

We're often sold the idea that we need to rid our body of toxins, particularly at certain times of the year like post-Christmas when "detoxing" becomes a buzzword. These "cleanses" might be in the form of juicing, fasting, drinking detox teas or taking expensive supplements. None of these have been scientifically proven to rid our body of toxins; our liver and kidneys already do that very efficiently on their own. Worse still, some of these approaches can be harmful. Juicing or fasting is extreme and restrictive, whilst detox teas and supplements often contain laxatives or diuretics which can both dehydrate us and cause depletion of important minerals like sodium and potassium.

Drink plenty of water and by all means enjoy a green juice as part of a balanced diet – but don't believe that anything you consume will somehow turbocharge flushing out your system. Your gut will always thank you for eating a balanced diet rich in fibre, probiotics and prebiotics (more on p.33) but it doesn't need a cleanse.

Myth 6: Sugar in fruit is bad for you

Fresh fruit provides valuable vitamins, minerals and fibre, but there is often confusion around the fruit sugar it contains: fructose. Studies have found some links between high-fructose corn syrup and increased heart disease – but this artificial sweetener isn't the same as fructose in fruit. On the contrary, a diet rich in whole fresh fruit (and vegetables) reduces the risk of heart disease.

We should aim to eat five portions of whole fruit and veg a day (see p.74 for what a portion looks like). Fresh, frozen or canned count, although if it's canned, choose fruit in natural juice or water with no added sugar.

Juicing fruit removes its valuable fibre; instead, blend fruit whole in a smoothie with fibre-rich veg and other nutritious extras (see p.84). The sugar in fruit juice (not whole fruit) is also considered a free sugar – the kind we should limit, that's either added to food and drink or naturally found in sweet foods like honey.

Sugary fruit juice and dried fruit can cause tooth decay if consumed in excess – juice in particular because it's acidic; dried in particular because it coats teeth. It's easy to consume both excessively, too: you wouldn't eat five apples at once but that's how many fill one glass of juice. Similarly, drying fruit shrinks its size, meaning you're likely to eat more than you would whole.

This bar chart illustrates how much more sugar a 100-g serving of dried apple or juice contains versus the same amount of fruit whole:

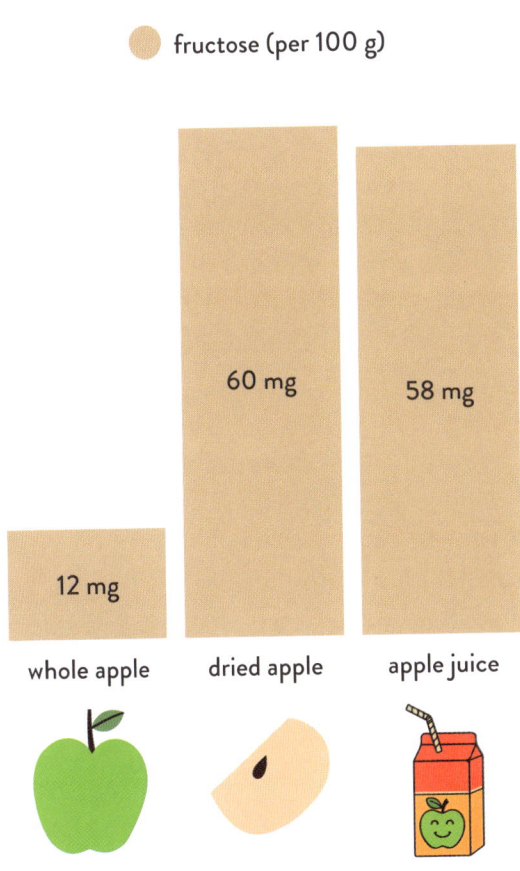

Myth 7: You should cut carbs to lose weight

If you follow a low-carb diet, such as keto, you'll likely lose some weight but it won't be sustainable in the long run, and studies show that these diets are hard to stick to. The initial weight loss might not be what it seems either. When we eat carbs, energy in the form of glucose is released into our bloodstream. Excess glucose is converted to glycogen and stored in the liver and muscles alongside water, at a ratio of one part glycogen to three parts water. If we cut carbs, we store less glycogen and therefore much less water with it. It's the loss of this water, not body fat, that causes much of the initial weight loss you might see on the scales.

Carbohydrates are our main source of energy, and restricting them may cause headaches, fatigue, low mood, poor concentration and constipation. But not all carbs are created equal. Refined carbs like white bread provide energy but have had the goodness of grains stripped away during processing. By contrast, wholegrains, as well as beans, pulses and vegetables, are healthier because whilst being a great source of energy, they also supply us with valuable nutrients such as vitamins, minerals – and fibre. Fibre greatly benefits our gut, and fibre-rich complex

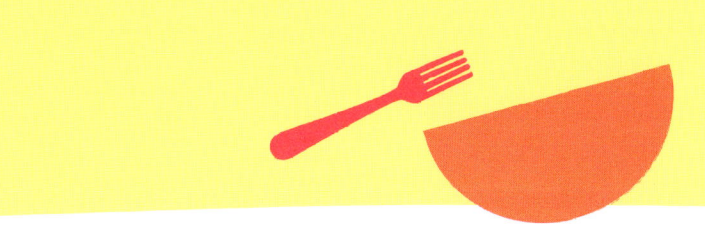

carbohydrates also give us a slow-release, stable source of energy because they take longer to digest than refined carbs. So, to maintain a healthy weight, in place of NO carbs, think SLOW carbs.

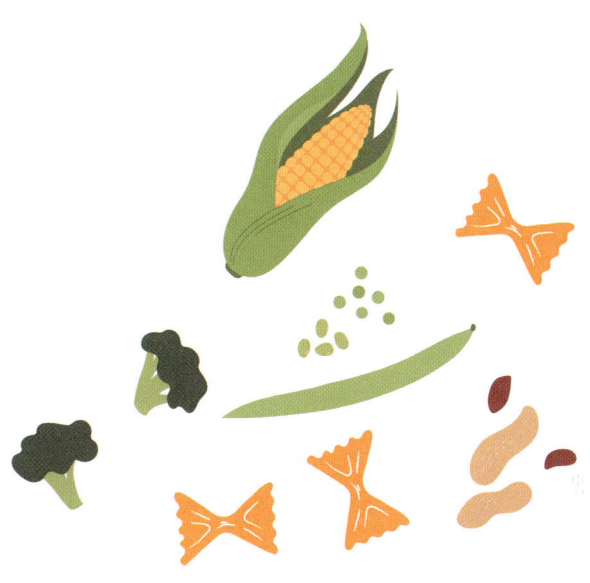

Myth 8: All cholesterol is bad

Did you know that cholesterol doesn't only come from your food – your body produces it, too? We make some "good" cholesterol in the liver, which our bodies need to carry out functions such as building cells. Cholesterol is transported around the bloodstream via particles called lipoproteins, of which there are two types: high-density lipoproteins (HDL) and low-density lipoproteins (LDL).

For good health, we need to keep a higher ratio of HDL to LDL. HDL is "good" cholesterol. It protects us by carrying LDL away from our arteries to the liver for removal. LDL is "bad" because too much can be harmful, accumulating on the inner walls of our arteries over time and eventually limiting blood flow. This can result in heart disease and stroke. Replacing saturated fat with monounsaturated and polyunsaturated fat and eating lots of wholegrains and legumes can lower LDL cholesterol. Getting plenty of exercise, maintaining a healthy weight, not smoking and not drinking too much alcohol can also keep cholesterol within a healthy range.

Types of cholesterol

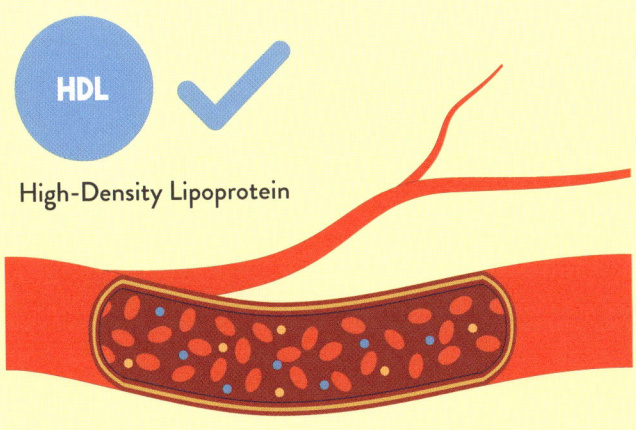

NORMAL ARTERY

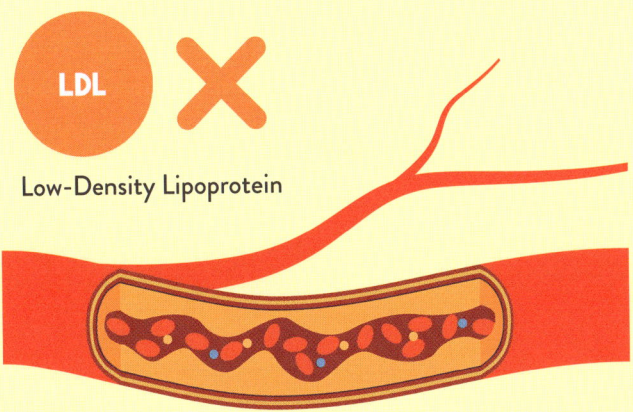

ARTERY NARROWED

Myth 9: Gluten is bad for you

There are many misconceptions about gluten. Some people must avoid it due to either a diagnosed allergy or coeliac disease. For these people, excluding gluten isn't a preference but a serious medical requirement – even a trace is damaging. For the rest of us, gluten does no harm.

Many foods that are naturally gluten-free, like vegetables or pulses, are also nutrient-dense. On the flipside, many high-in-gluten foods are also high in sugar, salt or saturated fat, such as pastries, pizza or battered fish. If we cut consumption of such foods in the name of going gluten-free, we will likely feel the benefit, especially if we eat more nutrient-dense wholefoods as part of the switch. But that doesn't mean the gluten itself is "bad" – we're simply making healthier choices and feeling better for it.

As any coeliac will tell you, eliminating gluten altogether can be extremely challenging. Gluten-free packaged goods are also expensive, so if you don't have to, you are needlessly overpaying. Don't fall for the idea that a gluten-free brownie is somehow a health food. A brownie containing sugar and butter is still a brownie, whether or not it's gluten-free.

Seek medical advice if you think you need testing for a wheat allergy, intolerance or coeliac disease (references on p.159). It's important you don't exclude gluten until after testing to avoid a false negative. And don't worry – if you do receive a positive diagnosis, you can still enjoy a delicious, balanced diet gluten-free.

Myth 10: You need protein supplements

Protein powders, bars and shakes are big business, but the truth is we don't need them. We can get all the protein we need from wholefoods (see p.18) with the benefit that these contain fibre, vitamins and minerals. Many high-protein products are manufactured with added oils and sugars, too, which mean extra calories.

For those of us who are active, eating a wholefood protein snack within an hour of hard exercise can aid recovery and repair muscle. Eat it alongside carbohydrates, like reduced-fat Greek yoghurt with a banana. If training hard, eat plenty of lean meat, fish, beans, pulses and lentils, and incorporate extra protein into your regular meals, like adding houmous to your usual sandwich.

Bear in mind that although protein repairs muscle after exercise, it's the exercise itself, particularly resistance training, that leads to muscle gain. Overdoing protein intake won't help because our bodies cannot store any excess. It'll be broken down and used for energy or stored as fat, not used to make bigger muscles.

Myth 11: All dairy is unhealthy

Unless you're vegan or you've been diagnosed with a dairy allergy or intolerance, there's no need to cut out dairy foods. They're excellent sources of protein, calcium, iodine, phosphorus, potassium and B vitamins. Some fermented dairy, like live yoghurt or kefir, also contains gut-friendly probiotics.

Dairy can be high in saturated fat so opt for lower-fat versions for day-to-day use, such as semi-skimmed or skimmed milk. Limit consumption of cream, butter and cheese. Dairy also contains a natural type of sugar called lactose which doesn't count as free sugar (see p.35) but some dairy products, such as flavoured yoghurts, can be sweetened with a great deal of added (free) sugar. Check labels and opt instead for reduced-fat, unsweetened and unflavoured Greek or natural yoghurt.

And, if you're vegan, ensure you include unsweetened plant-based dairy alternatives that are fortified with calcium, iodine and B vitamins.

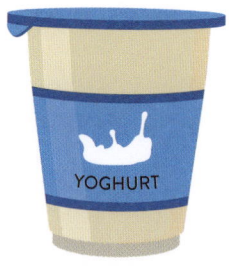

Myth 12: Baking with coconut oil and coconut sugar is healthier

Coconut oil gets touted as a "healthier" fat, but did you realize that it's a saturated fat? Moreover, per 100 g, coconut oil contains a greater amount (87 g) of saturated fat compared to 52 g in butter or 12 g in sunflower oil. As such, just like any fat in baking, it's best consumed in moderation.

Coconut sugar may also be marketed as "healthier", but it contains similar amounts of sugar (91 g) to 100 g caster sugar, and our bodies will treat both these free sugars equally. It's a similar story with other "natural" sugars: versus 100 g caster sugar, honey contains a little less at 80 g, agave contains 66 g and maple syrup 65 g – but all are free sugars, just the same.

Opting to bake with any sugar is personal preference, remembering that some might cost more at the checkout than others. Home baking is one of life's pleasures and certainly has its place in a balanced diet. Just don't fall for the myth that these "natural" ingredients make low-fat or low-sugar bakes.

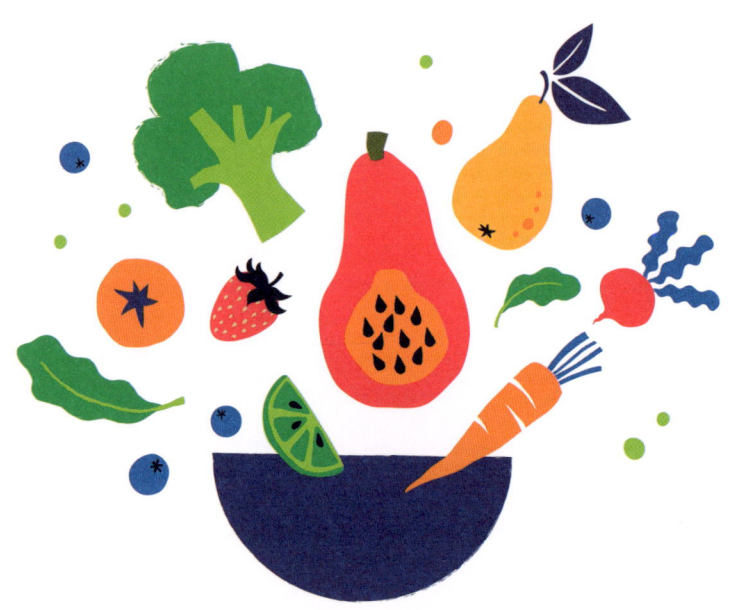

Chapter Three:
NUTRITION HACKS

Now you've read the theory, it's time to put the learning into practice. This chapter shares some hacks to help you enjoy a balanced diet, including simple food swaps and tips to prep fresh food quickly, effortlessly and on a budget. Learn to organize your kitchen, then get cooking with delicious, easy recipes for everyday eating.

What the heck is a hack?

These hacks are bite-sized tips that can help you get more nutrition into your meals every day. Dip in and out, try the ones that work for you or gradually adopt them all if they fit. But don't think you have to change everything all at once. Neither do you have to stop eating all your favourite foods. A balanced diet is about enjoying everything in moderation, so Hack Number One is eating a slice of chocolate cake if that's what you're craving today. Just perhaps cutting a smaller slice and serving it with some fresh berries and a dollop of yoghurt.

The recipes in this chapter are nutritious versions of foods we all like to eat: sandwiches, curries, pizza, pasta and cookies. These hacks aren't about restriction but instead about how we can modify our meals to make them more nutritious and boost our health.

Cook fresh, eat fresh

Preparing your own food gives you control of the nutrients you eat, and there's lots of evidence underscoring the benefits of regular home cooking: it can help you eat more plants, maintain a healthy weight and improve your sense of well-being. However, it's important to remember that the way you cook an ingredient can alter its nutritional value, so follow these tips to maximize health benefits:

- Season without salt and sugar
- Invest in an air fryer to minimize the amount of cooking oil you use
- Steam or blanch veg to preserve vitamin content, colour and texture
- Use non-stick cookware or baking parchment to avoid greasing, or use an oil spray or just a drizzle
- Sauté, stir-fry or griddle in place of shallow- or deep-frying
- Poach chicken or fish in broth in place of roasting
- Buy tinned foods with no added salt or sugar
- Make cheese go further by grating, not slicing
- Use low-salt stock

Straightforward food swaps

BREAKFAST

Swap...
- HFSS cereals
- Croissant
- Flavoured sugary yoghurts

For...
- Porridge or no-added sugar muesli
- Wholegrain toast with nut butter
- Reduced-fat plain Greek yoghurt with fruit

LUNCH

Swap...
- Savoury pastries
- Crisps/chocolate bar
- Soft drink

For...
- Salad/fresh soup/dip with veg sticks
- Unsweetened popcorn/trail mix (p.138)
- Water/unsweetened tea or coffee

DINNER

Swap...
- Red or processed meat
- HFSS jarred sauces
- White rice/pasta/noodles

For...
- Lean chicken/fish/plant protein
- Tomato sauce (p.118) and add vegetables to plate
- Brown rice and pasta/soba noodles

SWEET SNACKS

Swap...
- Biscuits
- Cake
- Sweet pastries

For...
- Chocolate-covered rice cakes/Medjool dates
- Energy balls (p.138)/brownies (p.142)
- Apple slices with nut butter/cookies (p.144)

NUTRITION HACKS

How to cut saturated fat, salt and sugar

Look back at the information on pp.35–37 and then try these hacks:

CUTTING SATURATED FAT:
- Swap full-fat milk in cereal, tea or coffee for semi-skimmed or skimmed and avoid creamy toppings on shop-bought coffee
- Switch pepperoni or ham on pizzas for chicken, tuna or veggies (p.118)
- Swap creamy pasta sauces for homemade tomato (p.118) or plant-based versions (p.120)
- Switch from coconut milk or cream-based curries to tikka (p.122) or a stir-fry (p.126)

CUTTING SALT:
- Season your food at the table with black pepper or chilli flakes instead of salt
- Buy low- or reduced-salt stock cubes, soy sauce, gravy granules, brown sauce, ketchup or baked beans

- Swap processed meat such as bacon, sausages, ham or salami for lean protein such as chicken, tuna or prawns
- Switch crisps for unsalted nuts and reduce the amount of salty cheese you eat by grating or crumbling it, or serving in small cubes or slices

CUTTING SUGAR:
- Cut sugar from tea and coffee and avoid syrups and sugary toppings on shop-bought coffee
- Switch jam, honey, marmalade or chocolate spread on toast for reduced-sugar spreads or nut butter
- Skip sweet and sour sauces. Use chilli flakes in place of sweet chilli sauce and reduced-sugar ketchup
- Peppermint or liquorice tea can ward off sweet cravings. Keep jars of bite-sized snacks to hand (p.138) as well

Easy ways to eat more plants

Aiming to eat 30 plants a week benefits both general and gut health. Fruit, veg, beans, pulses, legumes, nuts, seeds, grains, herbs and spices all count. Here are some simple ways to add more to your meals:

- Try meat-free Monday or cook sauces that are 50:50 – half meat, and half pulses or veggies
- Start ragus and soups with a soffritto base – a mix of chopped onion, garlic, celery and carrot (which you can keep in the freezer – see p.87)
- Add different colours to every plate
- Cook with dried herbs and spices
- Garnish with fresh herbs or chopped chillies
- Sprinkle nuts and seeds on salads, soups, porridge, yoghurt and smoothies
- Use pouches of mixed grains or jarred peppers and olives in salads
- Dollop tomato salsa or herby pesto (see p.98) on salads
- Add sautéed greens to mashed potato
- Add gut-loving kimchi or pickles to sandwiches
- Make dressings for noodles or salads with citrus and tahini (p.96) or miso (p.136)

Swapping refined carbs for plants

Refined carbs like white bread and pasta provide energy but have had the goodness of grains stripped away during processing. Replacing them (either partially or fully) with plants provides valuable vitamins, minerals and fibre, not to mention extra flavour and colour. Try these ideas for starters:

- Swap toast soldiers for sprouting broccoli or asparagus spears to dip in boiled eggs
- Switch white pasta for red lentil or pea pasta
- Serve finger foods in lettuce leaf wraps instead of tortilla wraps
- Mix standard spaghetti with courgetti noodles
- Add nuts and seeds to salads for crunch (see p.114) in place of croutons
- Substitute crackers or breadsticks for oatcakes
- Use creamy cannellini beans as you would risotto rice – ready in half the time, too! (ideas on p.124)
- Try cauliflower rice or quinoa in place of couscous
- Bake with ground almonds or oat flour (p.140) in place of white flour
- Swap lasagne sheets for sliced butternut squash

Ways to get more fibre

We should aim for 30 g of fibre a day, but the average intake is more like 18 g. So what does 30 g look like?

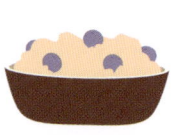 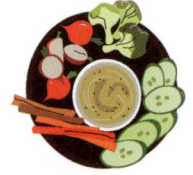 

PORRIDGE
- oats — 4 g
- banana — 1 g
- berries — 1 g
- chia — 1 g
- nut butter — 1 g

HOUMOUS LUNCHBOX
- houmous — 3 g
- granary bread — 5 g
- carrots — 1.5 g
- pepper — 1.5 g
- mange tout — 1.5 g

VEGGIE RAGU
- carrots — 1 g
- lentils — 3.5 g
- wholewheat spaghetti — 2 g
- a handful of unsalted nuts — 3.5 g

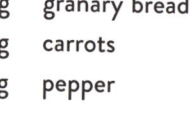

30.5 G

Other examples of high-fibre foods include two slices of wholemeal bread (7 g), a baked potato including the skin (7 g), a portion of reduced-salt baked beans (7 g) or a little bowl of edamame (8 g). Particularly high-fibre fruit and veg include dried apricots, berries, apples, broccoli, Brussels sprouts, cabbage, corn, green leafy veg, peas and sweet potatoes.

Flavouring food without sugar and salt

There are so many ways to add flavour without using sugar or salt; some ingredients can enhance both sweet and savoury dishes, as the diagram below illustrates. You'll find many of the flavourings below featured in the recipes later in this chapter. The internet is also a brilliant free resource – just search for an ingredient and browse for endless recipe inspiration:

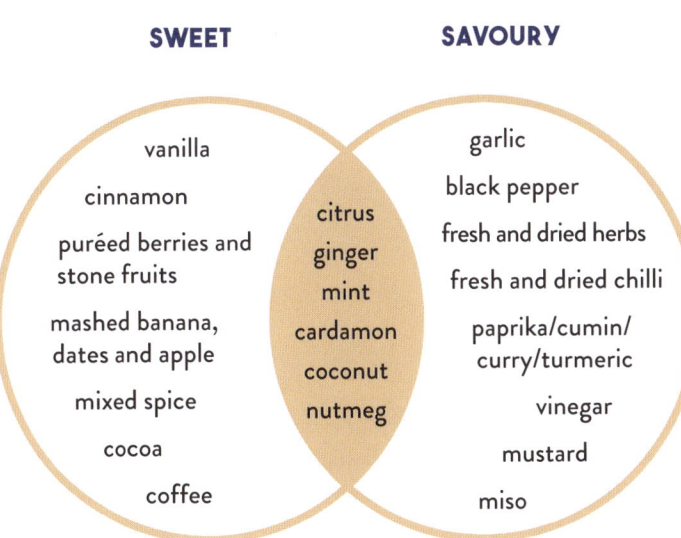

SWEET
- vanilla
- cinnamon
- puréed berries and stone fruits
- mashed banana, dates and apple
- mixed spice
- cocoa
- coffee

Both
- citrus
- ginger
- mint
- cardamon
- coconut
- nutmeg

SAVOURY
- garlic
- black pepper
- fresh and dried herbs
- fresh and dried chilli
- paprika/cumin/curry/turmeric
- vinegar
- mustard
- miso

Eyeballing portions of food

Portion control is a simple hack that can help us maintain a healthy weight. It's easy to eat bigger portions of food than our body needs but it can be tricky to know what size portion is about right. Take the guesswork out of it by using your hand as a rough measure. Serving food on smaller plates and eating mindfully (see p.41) can also help us eat appropriate-sized portions.

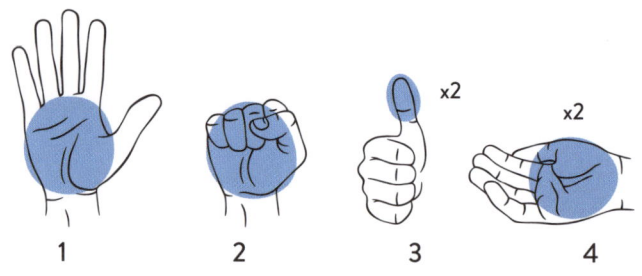

ONE-PORTION EQUIVALENTS

1	Protein e.g. chicken breast/scrambled eggs	Size of your palm
2	A serving of fruit or vegetables	Your clenched fist
3	Fat e.g. piece of cheddar cheese	Two thumbs together
4	Carbohydrates e.g. dried pasta shapes or rice	About two cupped handfuls

Staying hydrated

As part of a balanced diet, we should drink no fewer than 6–8 glasses (or 1.5–2 litres) of fluids a day. Water, sugar-free drinks and semi-skimmed/skimmed milk all count, as do tea and coffee without added sugar. Here are some simple tips to help you drink more:

- Get a reusable water bottle to keep track of how much you're drinking
- Try sparkling water, or flavouring still water with sliced citrus or cucumber
- Drink water with every meal
- Take your water bottle out with you during the day
- Set reminders on your phone or use an app to nudge you
- Drink regularly throughout the day
- Eat foods that are high in water such as cucumber, watermelon, strawberries, oranges, celery and tomatoes, as these also contribute to hydration

Caffeine

Caffeine is a stimulant, and some people are more sensitive to it than others. Moderate intake is around 300–400 mg a day. An excess can trigger symptoms including stomach upsets, and when consumed later in the day, caffeine disrupts sleep. Energy drinks are both caffeinated and often high in sugar. You can reduce your intake of caffeine by switching to decaf or trying different fruit or herbal teas instead.

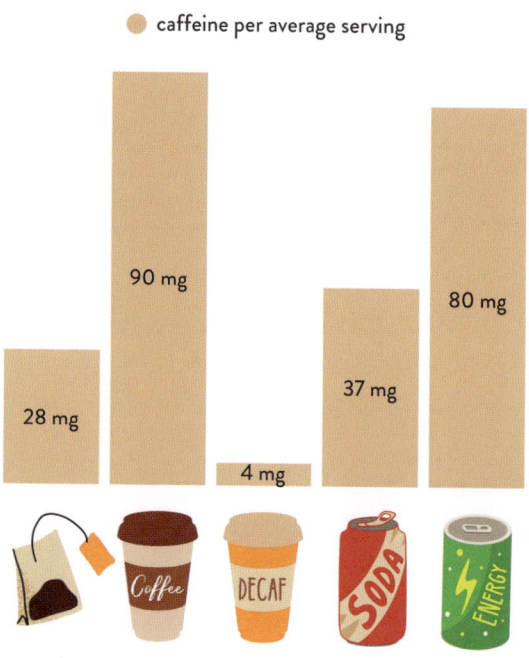

Alcohol

If you drink alcohol, you're advised to have no more than 14 units per week. Long-term drinking above these limits can lead to serious illness including heart and liver disease or cancer and may negatively impact mental health, whilst also causing weight gain. The less you drink, the lower any health risks. The units per drink depend on its strength and size. Below is an approximate guide.

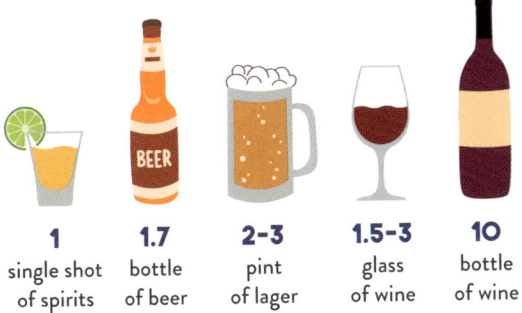

| **1** | **1.7** | **2-3** | **1.5-3** | **10** |
| single shot of spirits | bottle of beer | pint of lager | glass of wine | bottle of wine |

If you'd like to moderate your drinking, these tips can help:

- Try to have alcohol-free days each week
- Drink with food, not on an empty stomach
- Longer drinks like white wine spritzers can make the same number of units last longer
- Drink water alongside every alcoholic drink

Cutting down, or cutting out, alcohol has many benefits including improved sleep, energy, immunity and mood.

Superfast nutrition

The trick to adopting habits that stick is ensuring they're achievable and sustainable in the long term – a big part of that for most of us is time. These hacks help add extra nutrients every day, even when you're busy.

5-MIN PREP-AHEAD BREAKFASTS

Overnight oats	p.102
Smoothies	p.84
Avocado jars for toast	p.98

SPEEDY ON-HAND SNACKS

Trail mix	p.138
Energy balls	p.138
Crunchy seed mix	p.114

READY IN 15 MINS OR LESS

Miso and salmon soup	p.136
Sandwiches	p.92
Avocado pesto	p.98
Stir-fries	p.126
Dishes with tinned fish	p.130
Waffles	p.108

DOUBLE DINNER RECIPES FOR LEFTOVERS NEXT DAY

Meals with beans and pulses	p.124
Dips	p.116
Soups	p.112

Nutrinomics

Ingredient swaps to help you save

PROTEIN

red meat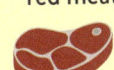

eggs

pulses and legumes

fresh fish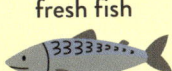

frozen and tinned fish

FRUIT, VEG AND HERBS

fresh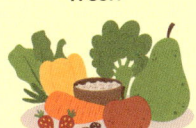

frozen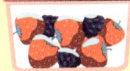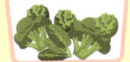

dried herbs

wonky veg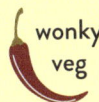

SUPERMARKET

convenience food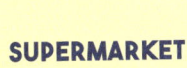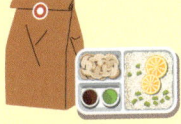

tinned tomatoes, beans and pulses

dried pasta, rice and noodles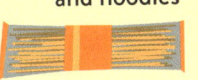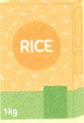

Eating well on a budget

Eating freshly prepared food is better for your health and tends to be more filling than fast food. This means you'll spend less satisfying your appetite. Check out the money-saving ingredient swaps you can make on p.79 then apply these tips to save money whilst shopping:

- Write affordable meal plans (see p.156) and shopping lists according to the ingredients you already have at home
- Sign up to supermarket loyalty schemes
- Consider using discounted ingredients for batch cooking and freezing
- Buy One Get One Free offers are only cost-effective if you wanted the food in the first place and if you know you can cook it all before the expiry dates
- Shop online to avoid being upsold extra goods in-store – you can also compare total prices in several virtual baskets before purchasing
- Buy own-brand supermarket goods and shop in discounted stores
- Shop at markets and greengrocers for better value fruit and veg
- Follow food bloggers who post low-cost recipe tips for free (but still be aware of being upsold fads you don't need!)

Eating well for the planet

Alongside our own nutritional needs, it's becoming ever-more important to consider the impact of our food choices on the environment. We can all take steps to eat in a more sustainable way for the sake of the earth's resources and future generations. These tips can cut the carbon footprint of foods you eat (and many will save you money, too):

- If you eat meat, consider reducing red meat to one portion a week or less and buying higher welfare
- Prioritize plant-based proteins in your diet in place of animal proteins
- Eat more local and seasonal produce if feasible
- Microwaves and air fryers use less energy than ovens
- Buy MSC-certified fish
- Recycle, reduce single-use plastic packaging and drink tap water, not bottled
- Reduce consumption of air-freighted foods and consider food miles
- Eat fewer takeaways and ready meals to reduce food packaging
- Compost food waste and grow your own herbs and veggies
- Support sustainable or B Corp food brands and restaurants

Forming lasting little habits

When it comes to our health, introducing small habits gradually can be more effective than trying to switch up everything at once. Making one positive change in our routine often snowballs into further healthy behaviours, too. Introducing an alcohol-free evening might mean taking up a team sport in place of going to the pub, for example, which together might lead to improved sleep.

It can help to identify your personal barriers to healthy eating then find ways to overcome them. For example, if you often feel too tired to cook dinner from scratch, try meal-prepping ahead when you do have more energy. Or if you find sticking to a plan and a budget difficult, try withdrawing your weekly food budget in cash at the start of the week, then challenging yourself not to spend extra on impulse food purchases.

7 steps for easy meal planning

Meal planning can help you stick to healthy eating throughout the week and needn't be complicated if you follow this method. For three ready-made weekly meal plans (easy prep, speedy and affordable), see Chapter Four on p.151.

START — Keep your kitchen organized (pp.86–89) so you can easily see what needs using and what needs restocking

Check expiry dates on foods and plan to cook with these first

Plan upcoming meals around ingredients you already have and need using up

On days you'll be short on time: plan to eat batch-cooked meals you've pre-prepared. On days with sufficient time: cook from scratch or batch cook to replenish stocks of meals

Factor leftovers into your plan for days you know they'll be handy

Write a shopping list according to your final meal plan and stick to it at the supermarket

Keep quick-cook, long shelf-life, fallback options to hand for days the meal plan unexpectedly backfires

NUTRITION HACKS

Anatomy of a smoothie

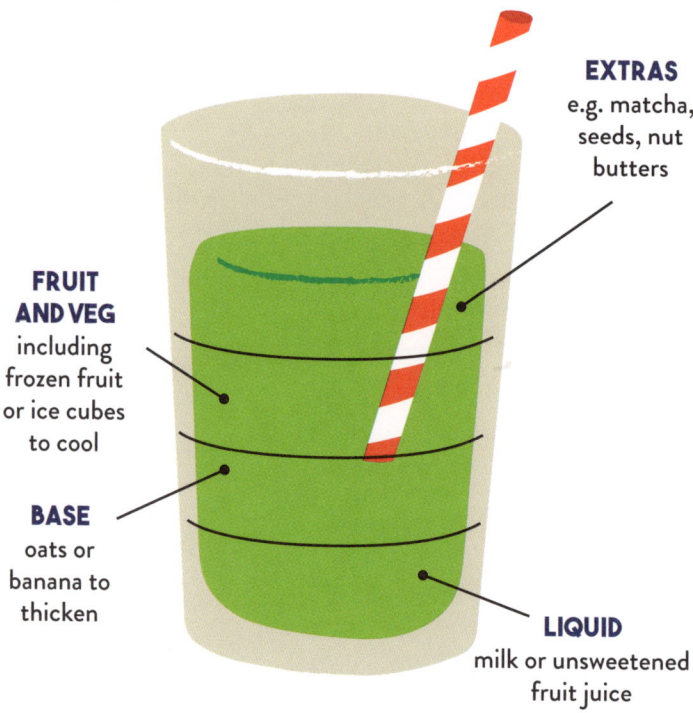

EXTRAS
e.g. matcha, seeds, nut butters

FRUIT AND VEG
including frozen fruit or ice cubes to cool

BASE
oats or banana to thicken

LIQUID
milk or unsweetened fruit juice

Smoothies are excellent for versatile, make-ahead or easy-prep breakfasts, as well as for quickly refuelling after exercise. Use whatever milk, fruit and veg you have on hand and keep bags of frozen fruit and oats on standby to throw in. Vary the little nutritional boosts you add with extras like seeds or nut butters.

Anatomy of a salad

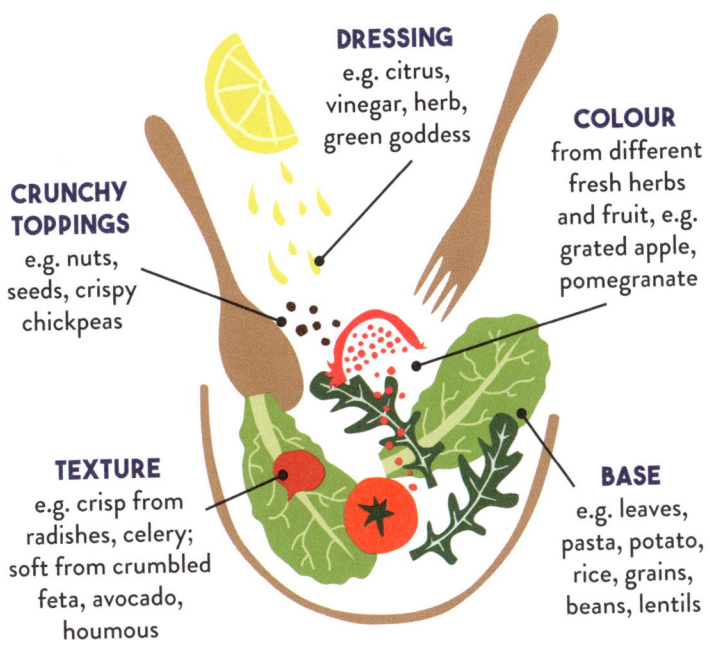

DRESSING
e.g. citrus, vinegar, herb, green goddess

COLOUR
from different fresh herbs and fruit, e.g. grated apple, pomegranate

CRUNCHY TOPPINGS
e.g. nuts, seeds, crispy chickpeas

TEXTURE
e.g. crisp from radishes, celery; soft from crumbled feta, avocado, houmous

BASE
e.g. leaves, pasta, potato, rice, grains, beans, lentils

Salads are endlessly adaptable and can be prepped ahead for lunchboxes or dinner. Make them into a more substantial meal by topping with cooked chicken, salmon or halloumi or by adding a side of sweet potato fries, (see p.134). Use whatever ingredients you have on hand and make up salad dressings (on p.96) ahead of time in the fridge. Add nutritional extras like nuts, seeds, grains, pulses and all manner of fresh and crunchy plants.

8 hacks for your fridge

Keeping your fridge organized speeds up meal planning, reduces food waste and saves you money. It's also important for food safety. Try these tips:

1. Keep fruit, veg and fresh herbs crisp in the salad drawers
2. Store raw meat and fish on the bottom shelf
3. Use dividers to group foods, such as yoghurts, with those that need using first at the front
4. Store prepared meals or ingredients in stackable plastic boxes or sealable bags, using a marker to label and date them
5. Prepare salads, grains or roasted veg in bulk and portion up for different days
6. Prep salad dressings ahead (see p.96) and store in screw-top jars – don't add to salad leaves until serving
7. Cook protein ahead e.g. chicken breasts, salmon fillets or boiled eggs to use in meals the next day
8. Prepare the following ahead to keep chilled: marinades (p.122), dips (p.116), overnight oats (p.102), smoothies (p.84), tomato sauce (p.118), salads (p.94) or peanut butter cups (p.146)

8 hacks for your freezer

A well-stocked freezer can be an emergency stash of economical last-minute meals. These standby ingredients all add flavour and nutrients – or are ready meals in themselves:

1. Freeze portions of soffritto – mixed chopped onion, garlic, celery and carrot – to use as the basis of soups and stews and up plant intake
2. Freeze fresh ginger or fresh chillies. You only use small amounts each time and both can be grated straight from frozen (no need to peel or deseed)
3. Keep bags of frozen fruits and vegetables to give all kinds of meals an instant plant boost
4. Frozen pre-prepped veg like butternut squash can save a lot of time
5. Freeze grated hard cheese to add straight to sauces or pasta
6. Turn old bread into breadcrumbs and freeze to add to pasta bakes
7. Freeze meals like chillies, ragus or soups flat in reuseable freezer bags that you can stack
8. Prepare the following ahead to keep frozen: bags of fruit for smoothies (p.84), green protein waffles (p.108), tomato sauce (p.118), meals with pulses and beans (p.124)

6 hacks for your kitchen cupboards

Keeping tabs on what's in your cupboards cuts down on food waste and means you always have nutritious ingredients available to cook with.

1. Use the first in, first out method by placing items you bought the longest ago towards the front of your shelves so that you use them first
2. Group similar goods together in containers (e.g. baking ingredients or dried herbs and spices) so that you always know what you have to hand
3. Stock up on wholegrains:
   - Brown rice, wild, black or red rice
   - Bulgur wheat and pearl barley
   - Oats
   - Quinoa and buckwheat
   - Spelt and farro
   - Wholegrain pasta
4. Keep supplies of tinned food:
   - Tinned tomatoes
   - Tinned tuna, crab and anchovies

- Black beans
- Cannellini beans
- Chickpeas and lentils
- Kidney beans

5 Buy unsalted nuts and seeds in bulk:
- Almonds, cashews, hazelnuts, peanuts, pecans, pine nuts, pistachios and walnuts
- Pumpkin, sunflower, sesame, poppy seeds, flaxseeds and chia seeds

6 Stock up on nutritious pantry staples:
- Monounsaturated and polyunsaturated oils (see p.22)
- Nut butter
- Tahini
- Condiments including vinegar and mustard
- Dried herbs and spices
- Miso

5 WAYS TO TOP A BAKED POTATO

All ready in 5–10 mins

Mix sweetcorn, chopped red pepper, coriander, finely sliced spring onion, lime zest and juice. Crumble over a little feta to serve. (Pictured.)

Mash drained tinned tuna with a dollop of yoghurt and stir in sliced radishes and celery, lemon zest and juice. Serve with mixed lettuce. (Pictured.)

Mix grated carrot with coriander, a pinch of cumin and a few pine nuts. Dress with a drizzle of olive oil and black pepper and stir together.

Scoop the flesh out of a baked potato and mash with a little steamed broccoli plus chopped chives. Spoon back into the potato skins, top with grated cheese and pop under a hot grill until the cheese is bubbling.

Make a slaw by mixing grated red or green cabbage, grated carrot, pumpkin seeds, lemon juice, olive oil and chopped flat-leaf parsley.

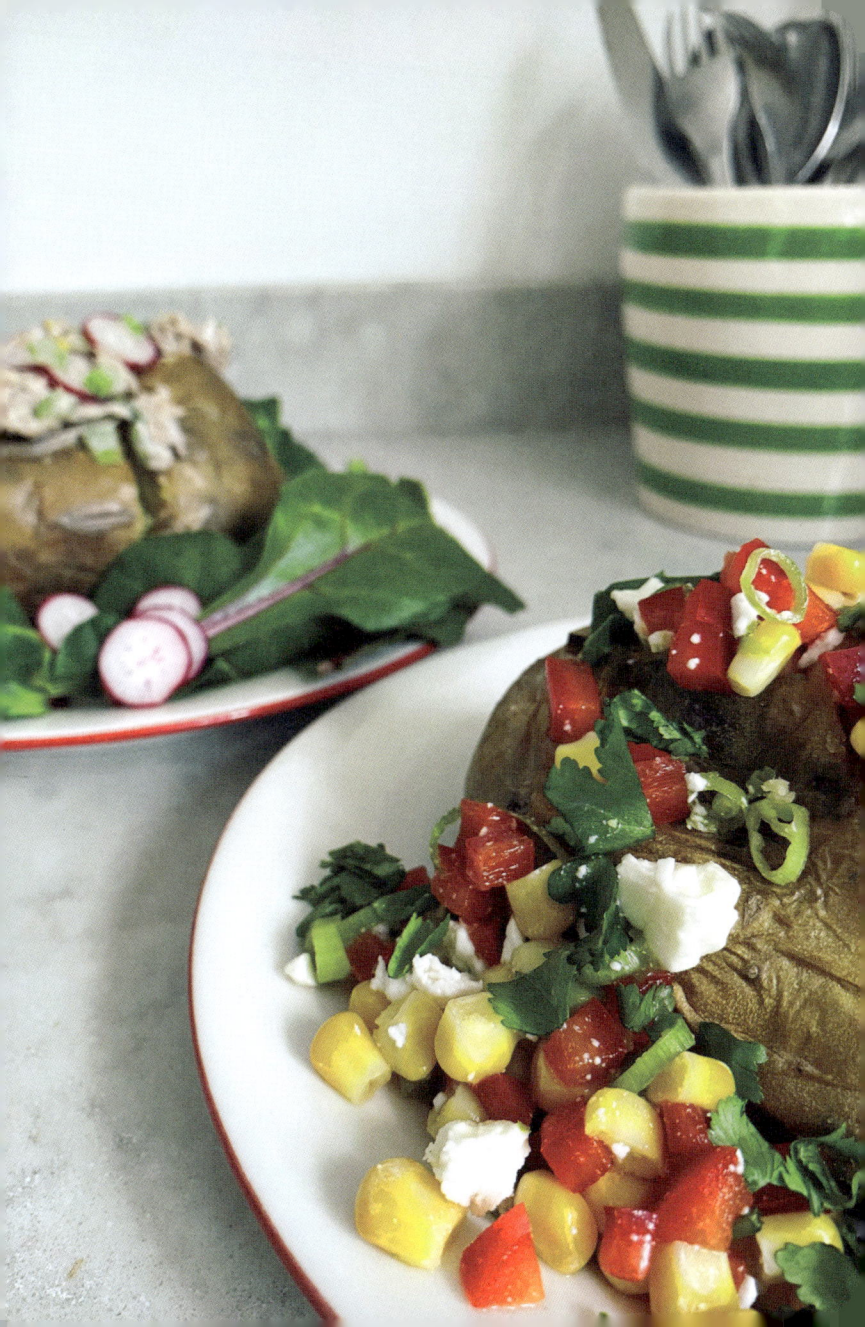

3 BALANCED SANDWICHES

All ready in 5–10 mins

Griddle a few slices of halloumi. Mix a little reduced-fat Greek yoghurt with shredded mint and spread over bread. Layer up the halloumi with sliced tomato and rocket.

Spread mashed avocado over bread. Mix shredded cooked chicken with reduced-fat Greek yoghurt, lemon zest and basil and layer up with green salad and cucumber.

Mix 2 tbsp reduced-fat Greek yoghurt with the juice of a lime, 1 tbsp mango chutney, 1 tsp each of curry powder and turmeric, plus plenty of chopped coriander. Stir in a drained tin of chickpeas. Layer up in a sandwich with sliced cucumber and shredded baby/Little Gem lettuce.

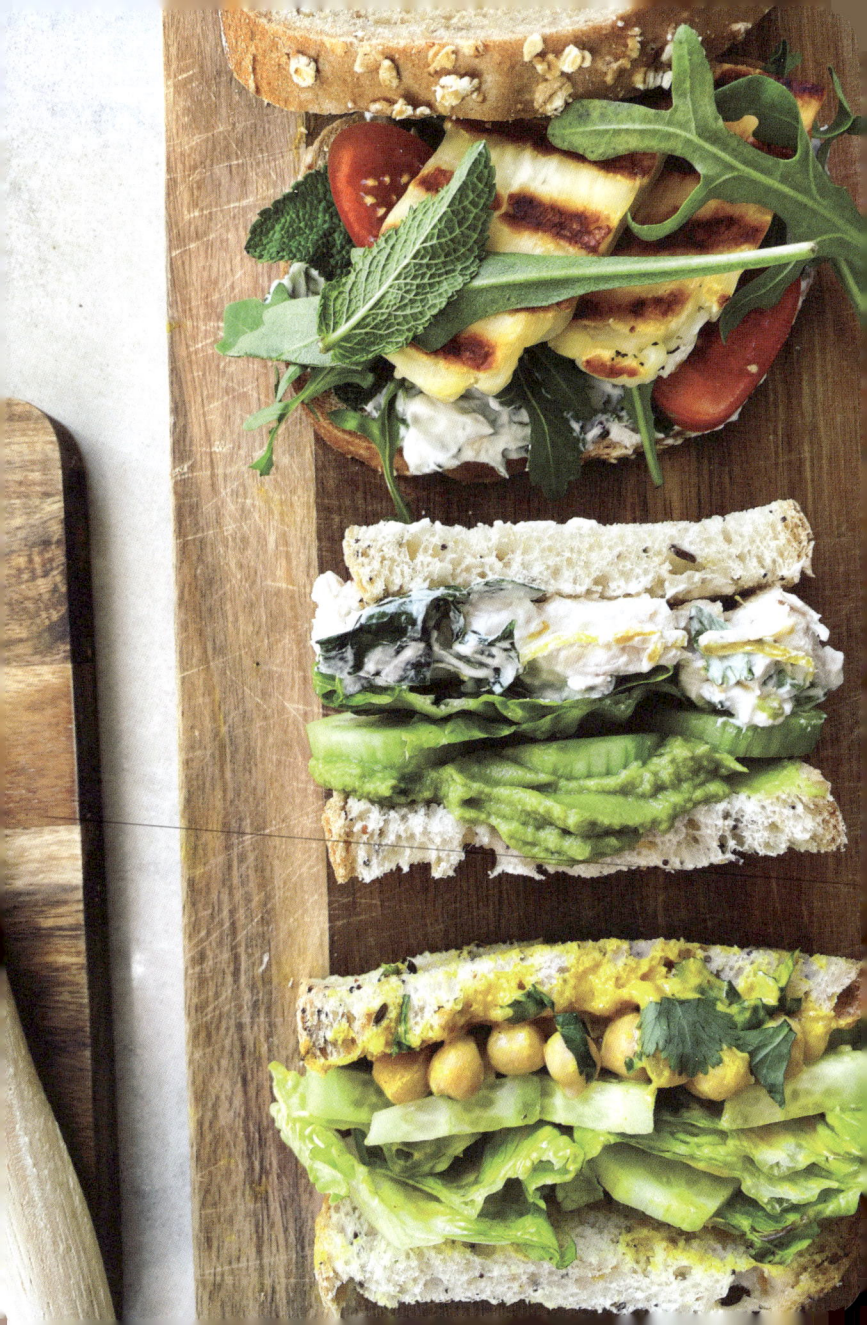

3 SUPERFOOD SALADS

All serve two | All ready in 20 mins or less

Dry-fry cubed halloumi in a pan. Meanwhile, cook 50 g buckwheat and 50 g quinoa for 10 minutes with a handful of frozen edamame and 80 g cut broccoli. Drain and mix with 2 sliced spring onions, half a diced green pepper and the halloumi. Dress with a little bright yellow dressing (see p.96) and top with toasted flaked almonds, chopped flat-leaf parsley and mint.

Preheat the oven to 220°C/200°C fan/gas mark 7. Mix cubed sweet potato, bite-sized cauliflower, crushed garlic and olive oil in a baking dish and cook for 15 minutes. In the final few minutes, add a baking tray of kale to the oven to crisp up (no oil needed). Add everything to two bowls with chopped avocado, pomegranate seeds, shredded cabbage, lettuce and beetroot houmous (p.116). Scatter with crunchy seed mix (p.114).

Steam green beans and/or sugar snap peas then mix with chopped roasted hazelnuts and orange zest. Add to plates with a drained tin of puy lentils, sliced baby tomatoes, mini mozzarella balls and shredded basil. Dress with a little chive vinaigrette (p.96).

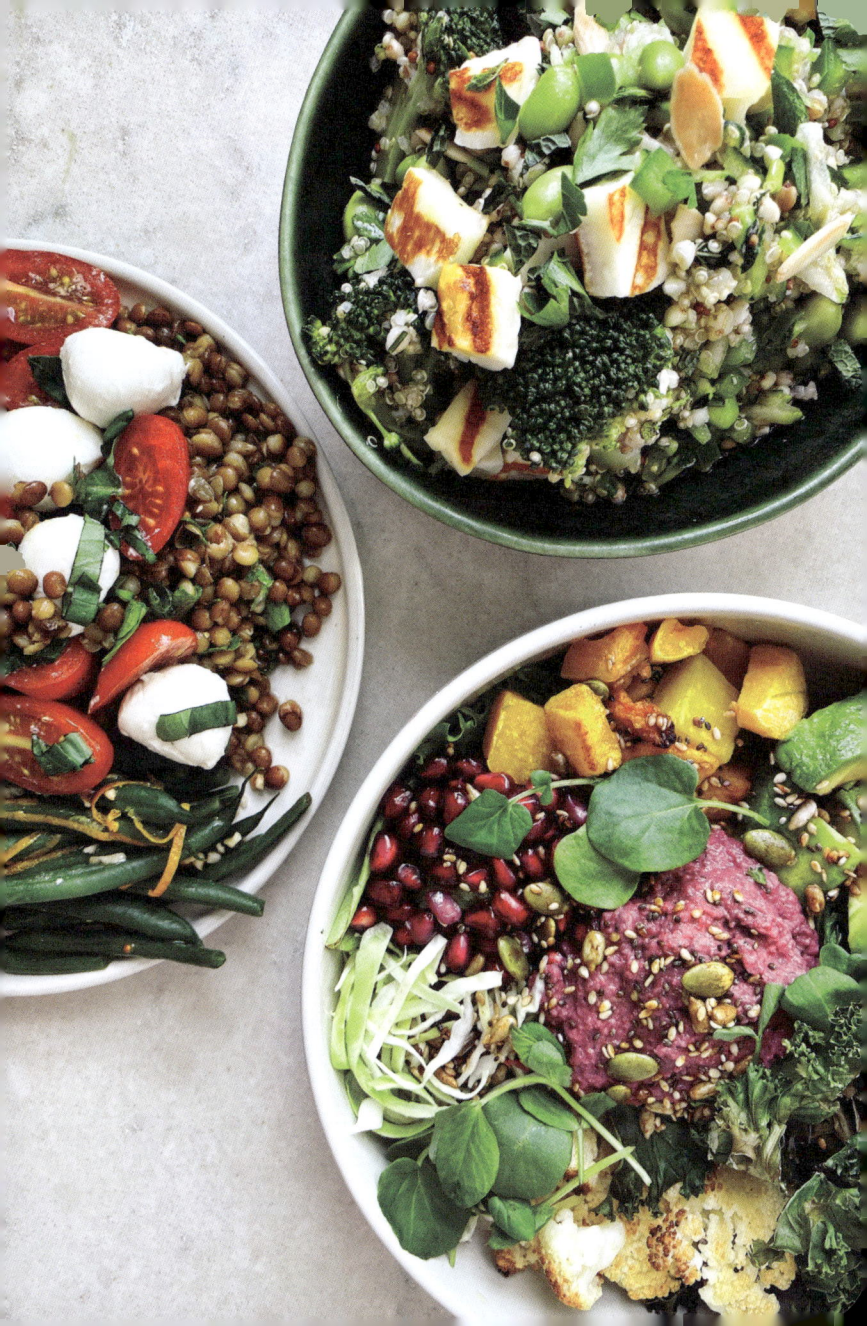

3 SALAD DRESSINGS

All make one jam jar (store in fridge) | *All ready in 5 mins*

Bright yellow dressing: Add half a crushed clove of garlic, the juice of a lemon, 25 ml rapeseed oil and 25 ml extra-virgin olive oil to a jam jar with a lid, close and shake.

Green goddess dressing: Add 2 tbsp tahini, 2 tbsp olive oil, the juice of half a lemon, 1 tsp honey, half a clove of garlic, 3 tbsp warm water and a good handful each of basil and flat-leaf parsley to a blender. Blitz until smooth.

Chive vinaigrette: Add 2 tbsp white wine vinegar, 1 tsp Dijon mustard, 1 tsp honey, 90 ml olive oil and 1 tbsp chopped chives to a jam jar with a lid, close and shake.

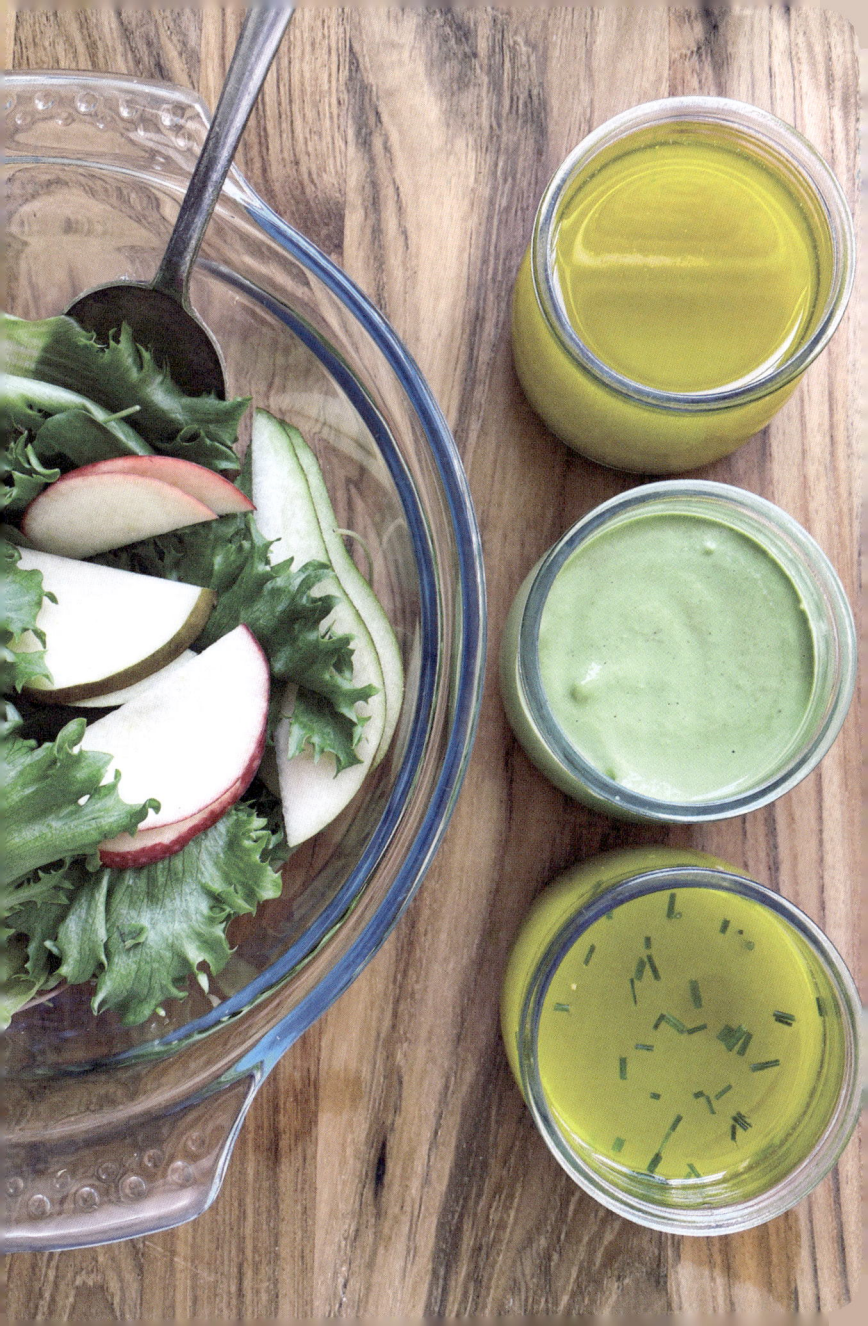

3 MEALS TO MAKE WITH AVOCADOS

All serve two | *All ready in 5 mins*

Make a silky green smoothie bowl by whipping an avocado in a high-speed blender with a handful each of baby spinach, frozen mango chunks and oats plus a small glass of semi-skimmed milk and 1 tsp honey. Blend until all the spinach is fully incorporated. Top with fruit and chopped toasted nuts (pictured) or seeds and granola (see p.100).

For a prep-ahead breakfast, use a fork to mash an avocado with a small tin of drained butter beans. Finely slice a little coriander and stir in along with the juice of a lime. Pop in a jar and spread on toasted sourdough the next morning.

Make avocado pesto by roughly blending an avocado with lemon juice, half a small clove of garlic, a little olive oil and plenty of basil. Stir through spaghetti topped with a little grated Parmesan and toasted pine nuts.

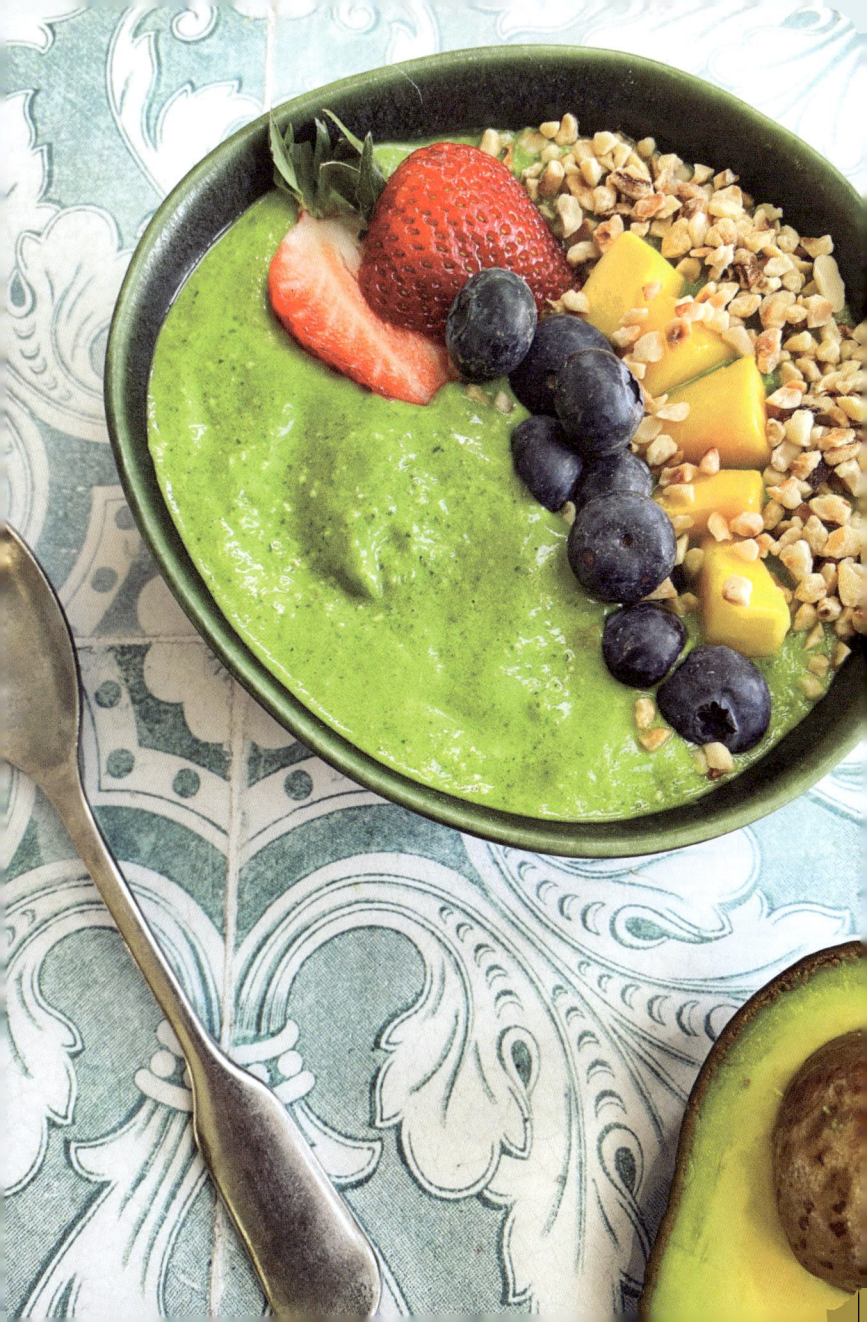

3 BIG-BATCH BREAKFAST CEREALS

All make a 1-litre jar | *All ready in 45 mins or less + cooling*

Muesli: Gently toast 200 g oats in a frying pan. Add 75 g chopped pecans and 100 g pumpkin or sunflower seeds and stir for another minute. Take off the heat and add a handful each of chopped dried apple and chopped dates. Leave to cool.

Granola: Preheat the oven to 150°C/130°C fan/gas mark 2. Mix 200 g oats with 75 g chopped pecans and 100 g pumpkin seeds, then stir in 75 ml honey, 60 ml sunflower oil, ½ tsp vanilla extract and ½ tsp ground cinnamon. Spread on a large, lined baking sheet and bake for 40 minutes, stirring halfway. Leave to cool.

Cocoa pops: Preheat the oven to 150°C/130°C fan/gas mark 2. Mix 75 ml sunflower oil, 50 ml honey and 3 tbsp cocoa into a large pan and heat for 2 minutes. Take off the heat and stir in 250 g buckwheat, 250 g quinoa, 75 g chopped cashews and 100 g sunflower seeds. Spread on a large, lined baking sheet and bake for 15 minutes. Leave to cool.

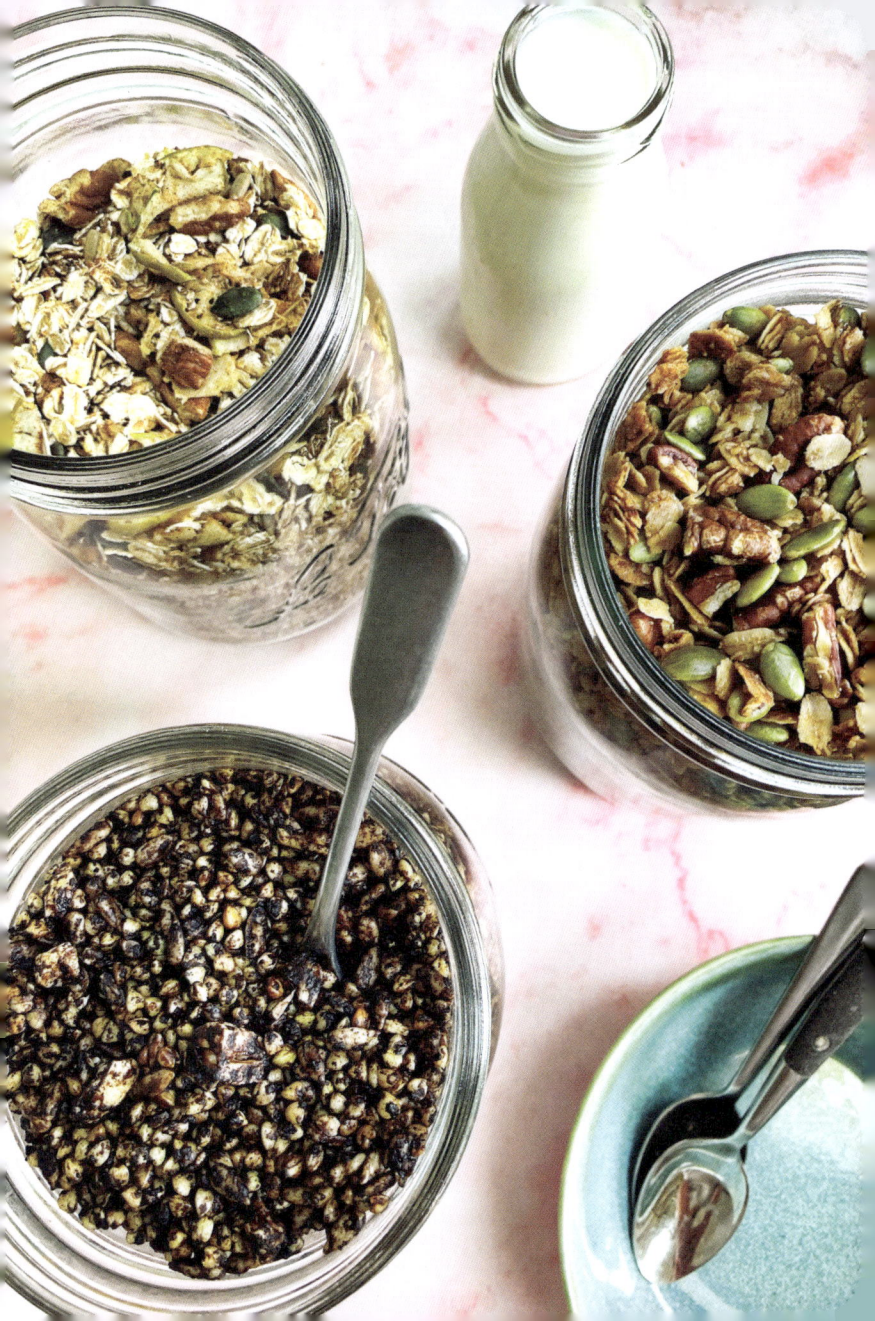

3 IDEAS FOR OVERNIGHT OATS

All make one small pot

All ready in 5 mins + chilling overnight in the fridge

Berry purée: Blend a handful of strawberries and raspberries. Add 1–2 tbsp muesli or granola to a jar and cover with a layer of reduced-fat Greek yoghurt then add a layer of berry purée. (Pictured.)

Carrot cake: Mix together a handful of oats, a little semi-skimmed milk, a pinch of cinnamon, 1 tsp chia seeds, a little grated carrot and a few raisins. Decant into a jar and top with a layer of reduced-fat Greek yoghurt and a few chopped pecans.

Blueberry and banana: Add a layer of oats to the bottom of a jar, pour in a little semi-skimmed milk, add a dollop of reduced-fat Greek yoghurt, a handful of blueberries and a small dollop of nut butter. Stir together and top with pumpkin seeds and sliced banana.

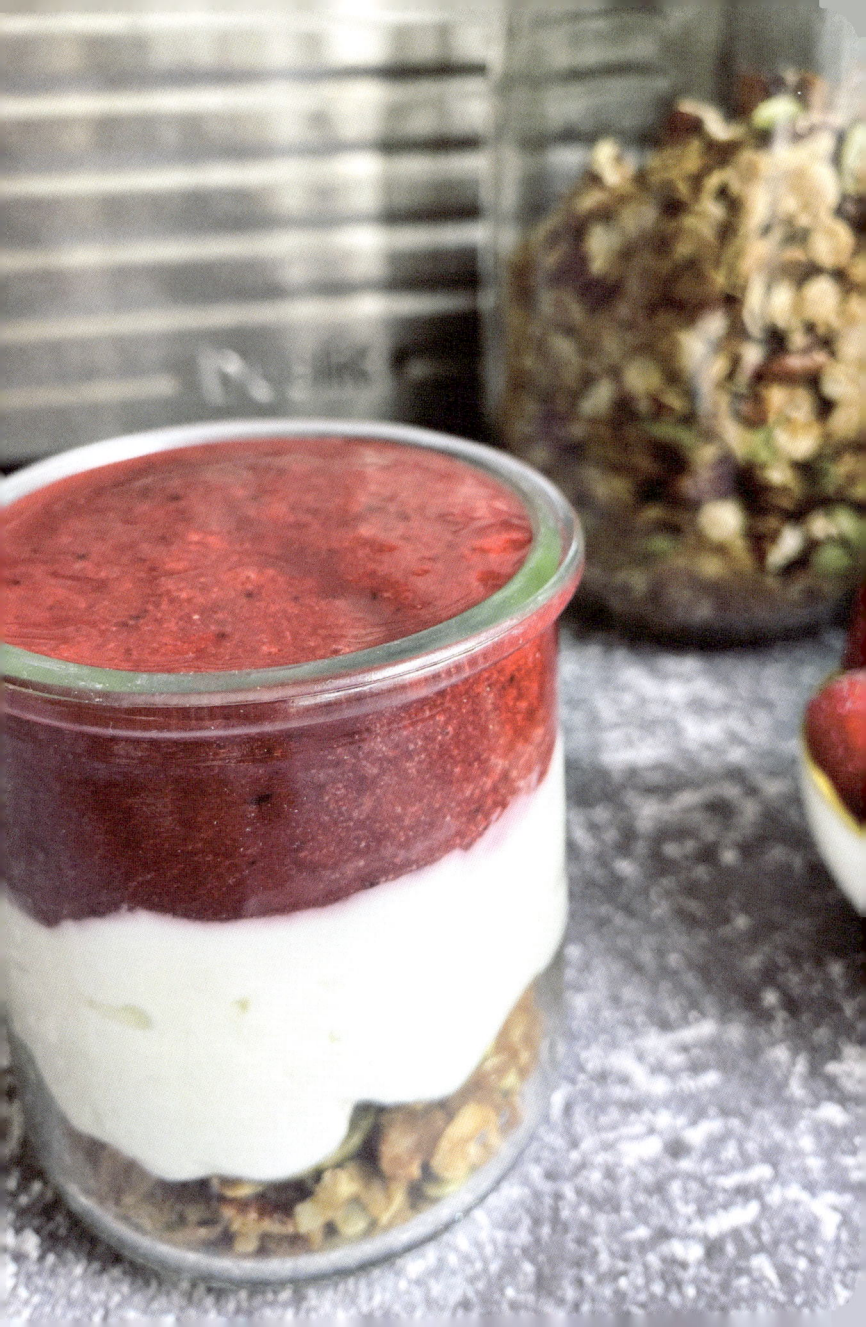

3 PROTEIN-RICH BREAKFASTS

All ready in 10 mins

Mix a little reduced-fat cream cheese with lemon zest and chopped dill. Spread on sourdough or seeded bread and top with smoked salmon, rocket and lemon wedges to squeeze over. (Pictured.)

Make breakfast tacos for a weekend brunch. Spread lightly toasted mini corn or wheat tortillas with mashed avocado, diced tomatoes and chopped coriander then top with scrambled eggs, chilli flakes or Tabasco, and a squeeze of lime. Or for a simple classic, whisk eggs with salt and pepper and gently scramble in a non-stick pan. Serve on toast with watercress.

Add a handful of quinoa to your normal porridge oats, cook with your choice of milk then top with peanut butter, reduced-fat Greek yoghurt, chopped nuts and seeds – all these ingredients are good sources of protein. Finish with chopped fruit or compote.

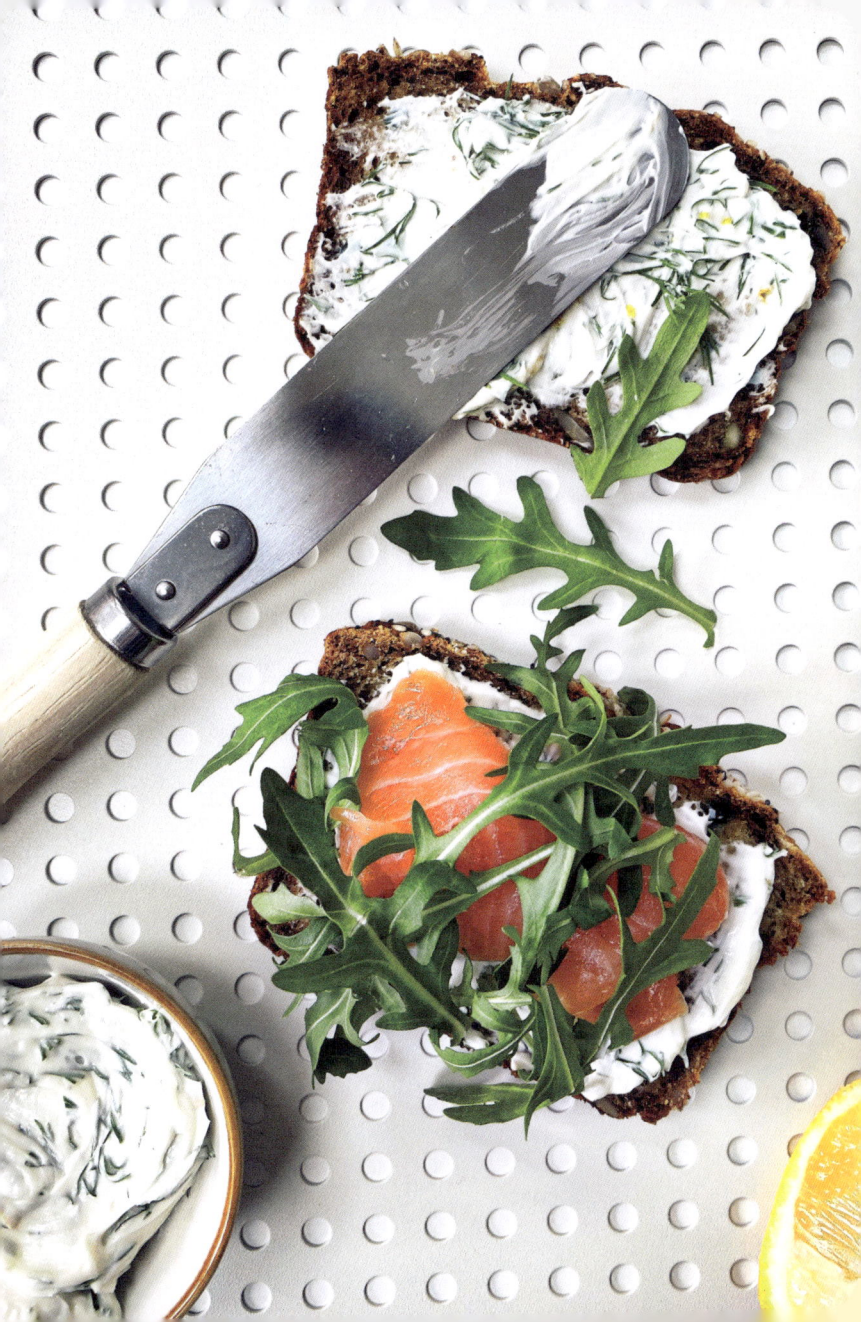

SEEDED OAT BREAD

This fluffy soda bread is very easy to make and excellent toasted – try freezing it sliced to toast from frozen as you go. Ensure your bicarbonate is fresh to get the best rise on your loaf.

Makes one loaf | *Ready in 1 hr 10 mins*

- 120 g oats
- 230 g plain flour
- 1 tbsp honey
- 75 g mixed seeds
- ½ tsp salt
- 2 tsp bicarbonate of soda
- 2 tbsp sunflower oil
- 500 g natural yoghurt

Preheat the oven to 180°C/160°C fan/gas mark 4 and line a 450 g (1 lb) loaf tin with baking parchment. Add the oats, flour, honey and most of the seeds to a large mixing bowl then sprinkle over the salt and bicarbonate of soda. Separately mix together the sunflower oil and yoghurt then tip into the oat mixture and stir everything together. Spoon into the tin, flatten the top slightly with the back of a spoon then scatter over the remaining seeds and gently press down with the spoon. Bake for 1 hour then turn out onto a wire rack to cool completely before slicing.

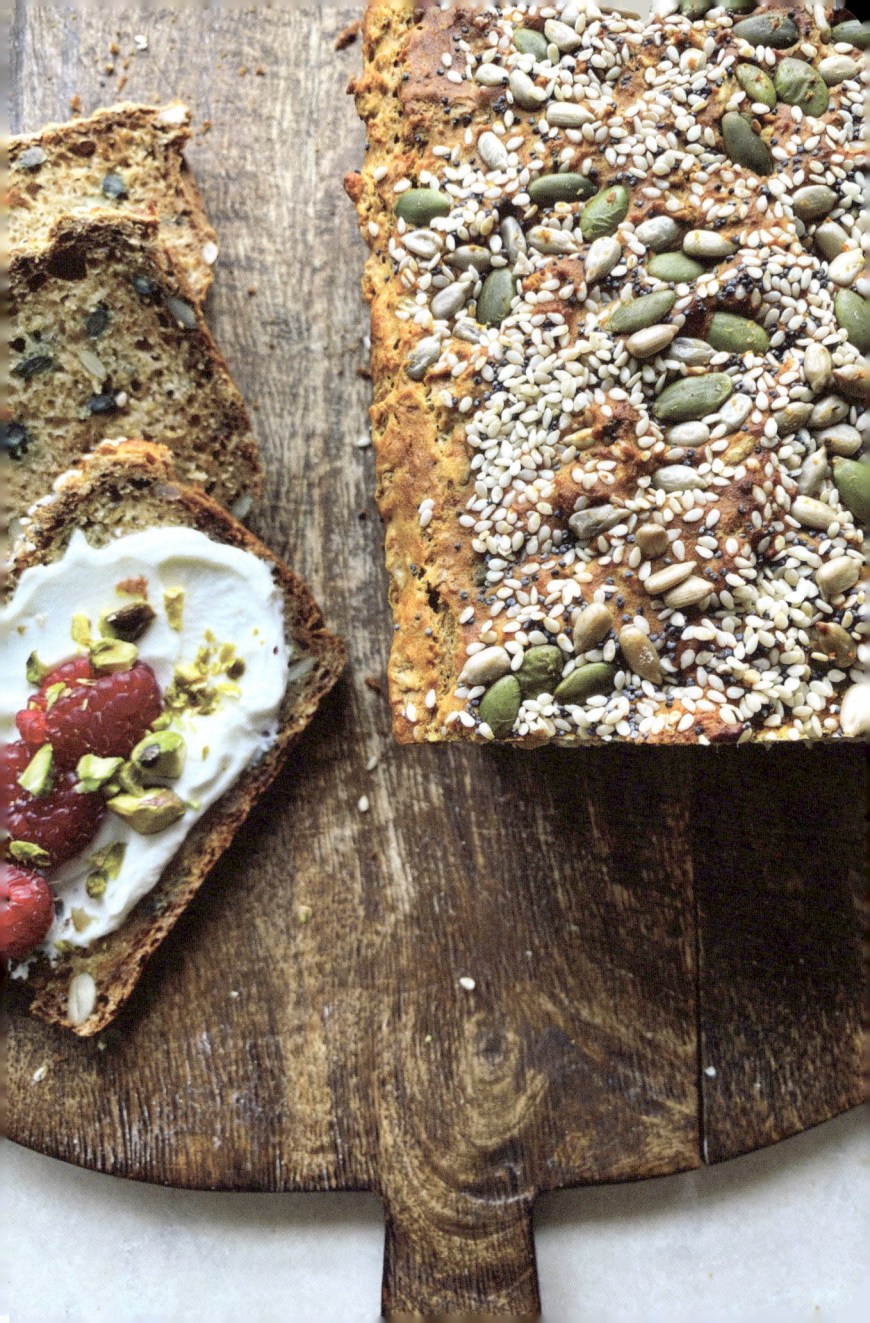

GREEN PROTEIN WAFFLES

These waffles are packed with protein from eggs, cottage cheese and oats. You can make them sweet or savoury according to the toppings you use and they're freezable so you can make a batch ahead and then quickly reheat one or two from frozen when you fancy them.

Makes 10–12 | *Ready in 10 mins*

- 300 g tub of low-fat cottage cheese
- 4 eggs
- oats
- 4 handfuls of baby spinach
- ½ tsp baking powder

Add the cottage cheese to a food processor with the eggs. Use the cottage cheese tub to measure out a full tub of oats and add these to the processor with the baby spinach and baking powder. Blend to a smooth batter and then cook in a waffle iron.

Topping suggestions on p.109, clockwise from top left: peanut butter and blueberries; reduced-fat Greek yoghurt and freeze-dried raspberries; guacamole (p.128) and pea shoots; beetroot houmous (p.116) and crunchy seed mix (p.114); tzatziki and mint; whipped butter bean dip (p.116) and rocket.

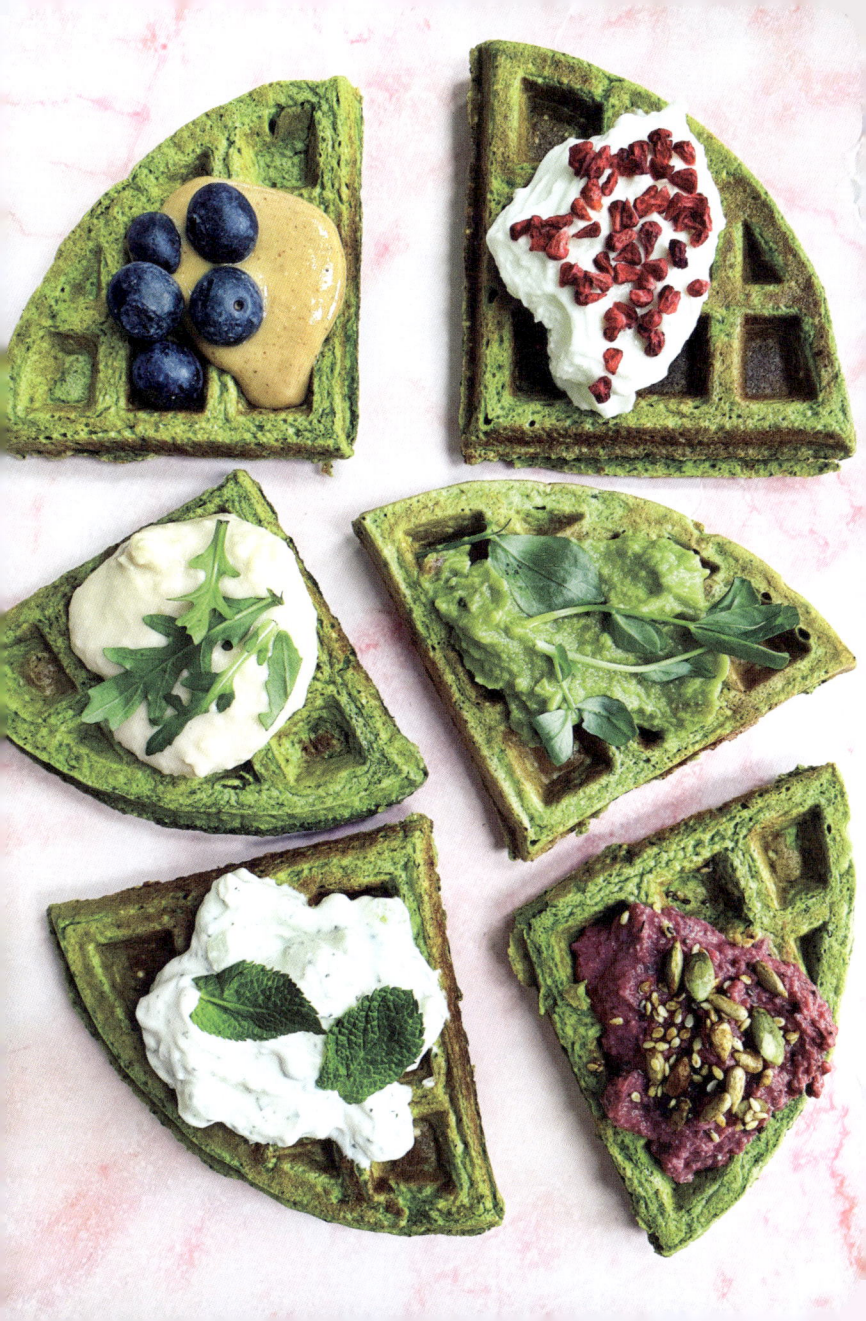

MATCHA SMOOTHIE

Here's an example smoothie made according to the blueprint on p.84. Matcha is a type of green tea from Japan. It's rich in antioxidants which help protect our cells from damage.

Makes one | *Ready in 5 mins*

- a small glass of semi-skimmed milk
- a handful of baby spinach
- 1 apple, quartered
- a handful of frozen mango
- 1 tbsp oats
- half a banana
- a squeeze of lime
- 1 tsp matcha powder

Blend everything together and serve.

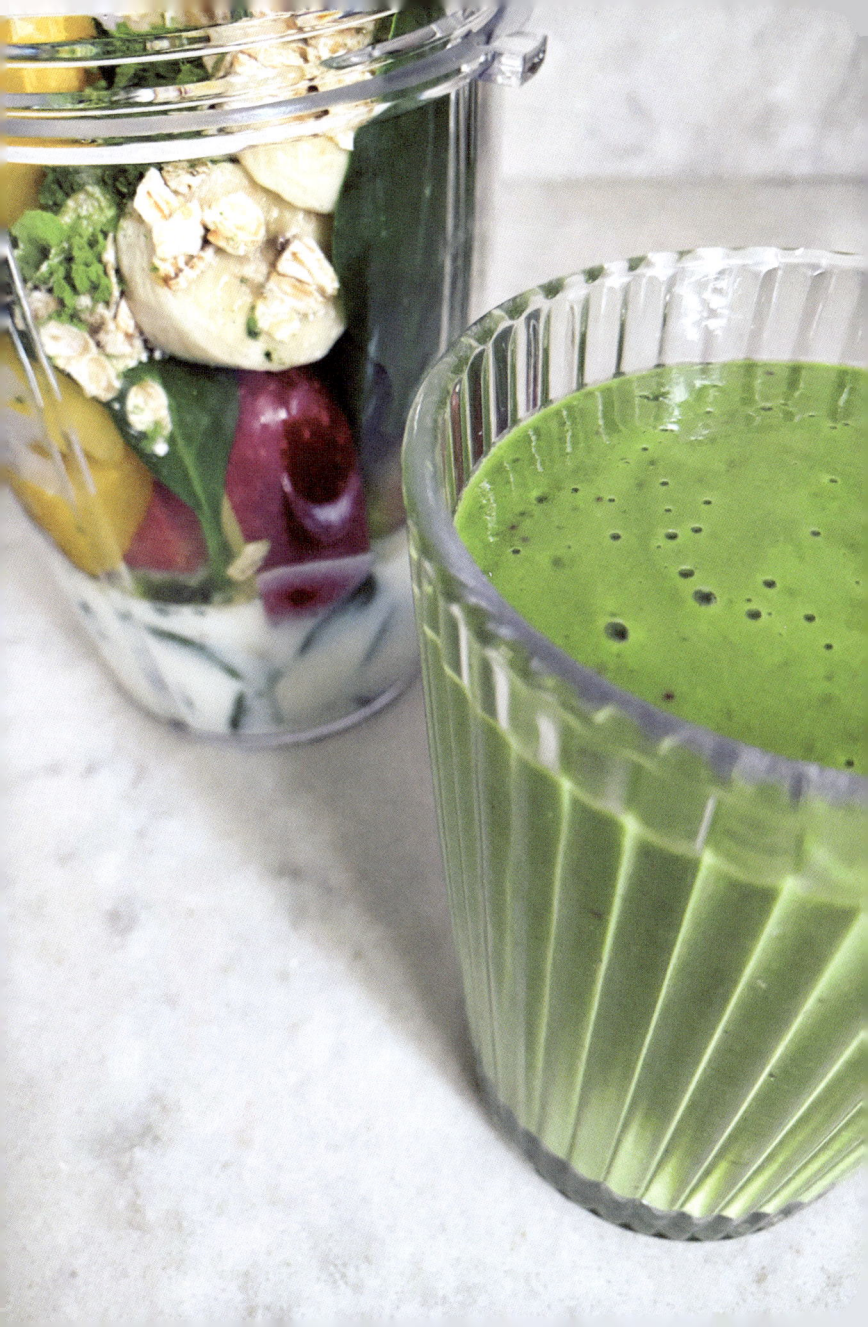

2 SIMPLE SOUPS

Both serve two | *Both ready in 20 mins or less*

Cheat's pho: Soften crushed garlic and grated ginger in a drizzle of sesame oil in a pan then add a handful of frozen prawns. Cook for 5 minutes then keep to one side. Add 500 ml low-salt stock to the pan with 2 small handfuls of jasmine rice. Simmer until the rice is cooked. Pour into bowls and top with the prawns, sliced spring onion, chopped chilli, julienned carrot, mint, coriander, basil and lime juice.

Tortellini soup: Soften a diced onion and crushed garlic in a pan with olive oil. Add a tin of tomatoes, fresh or dried thyme and 450 ml low-salt stock. Simmer for 10 minutes then blend until smooth. Return to the hob over a low heat, adding a pack of fresh tortellini to cook in the soup (about 3 minutes). Serve with grated Parmesan.

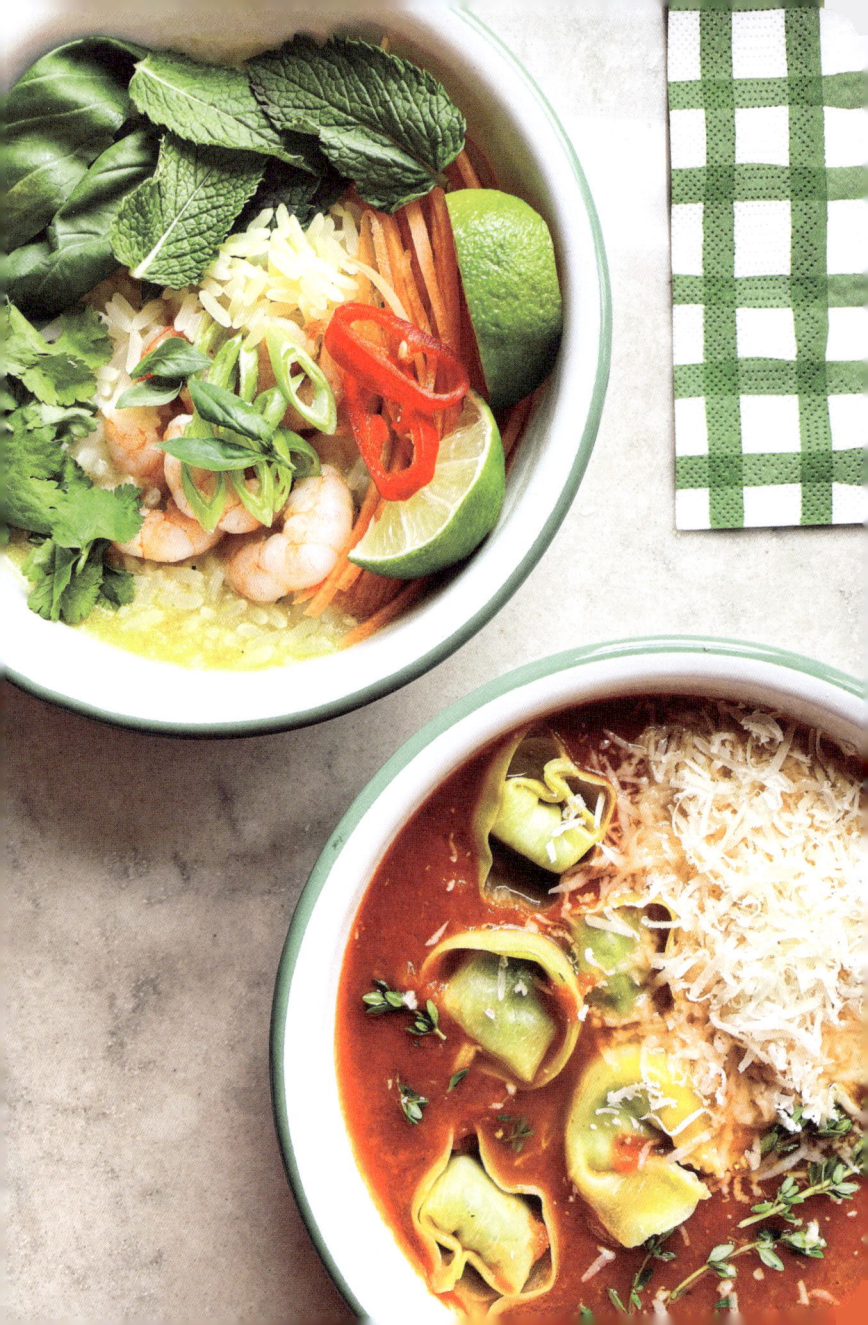

CRUNCHY SEED MIX

Makes one jar | *Ready in 5 mins + cooling*

Add 2 tbsp of each of the following to a large non-stick frying pan: pumpkin seeds, sunflower seeds, sesame seeds and chia seeds. Toast over a high heat for a few minutes, stirring so that they don't catch. Once the seeds start to pop and take on some colour, remove from the heat and immediately add 1 tbsp reduced-salt soy sauce. Mix, then leave to cool before transferring to a jar with a lid. Enjoy sprinkled over salads and soups (like the below) and eat within a month.

LEEK AND CANNELLINI BEAN SOUP

Serves two | *Ready in 20 mins*

Soften a sliced leek in olive oil with crushed garlic. Add 500 ml low-salt stock and a drained tin of cannellini beans. Simmer for 10 minutes, adding a handful of frozen peas in the final minute. Blend with a splash of semi-skimmed milk and 2 handfuls of basil. Top with crumbled feta and crunchy seed mix.

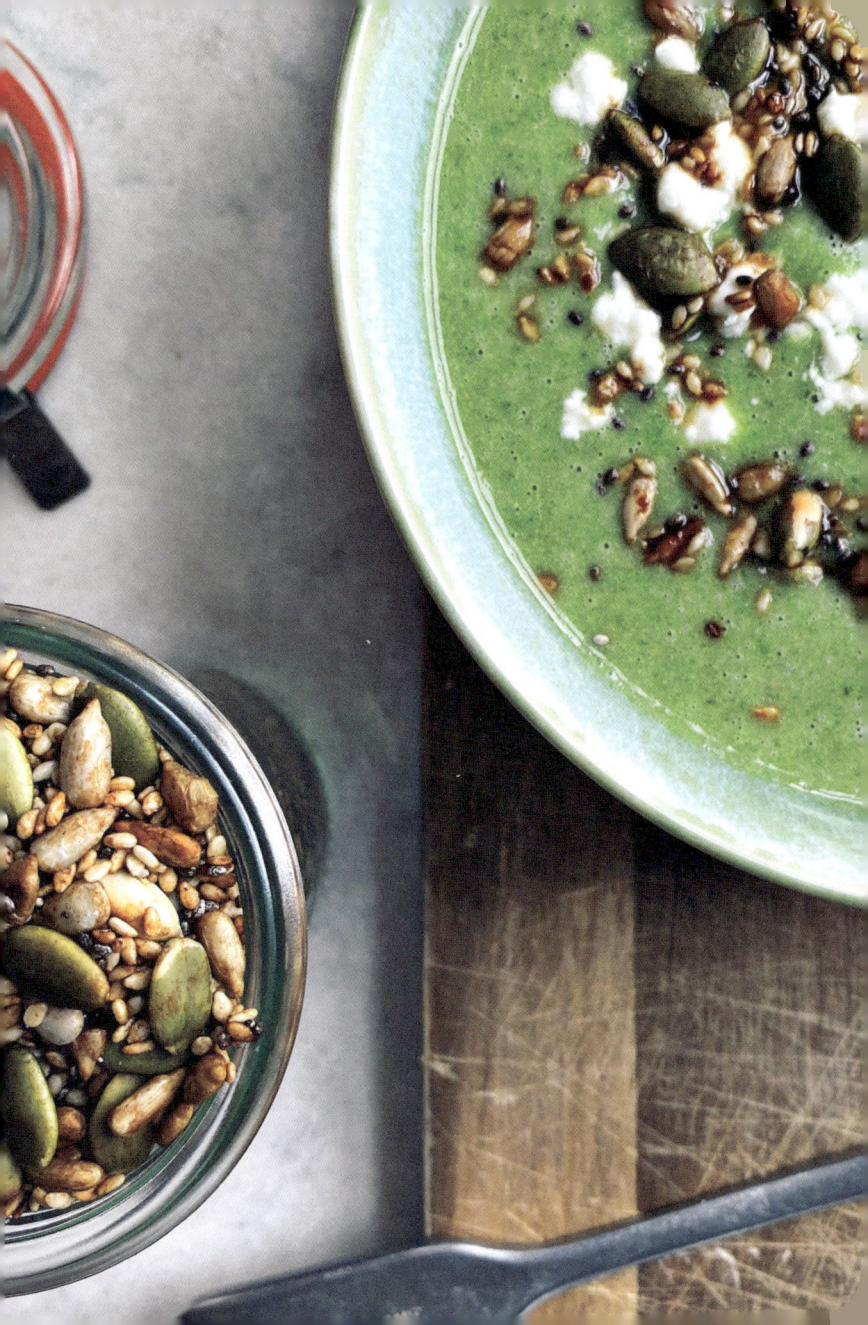

3 EASY DIPS

Serve these dips with chopped raw veg or oatcakes or you can dollop them onto the top of salads (suggestions on p.94).

All serve two | All ready in 5 mins

Whipped butter bean: Blend a drained tin of butter beans with 2 tbsp olive oil, a clove of garlic, the juice of a lemon and 1–2 tbsp water to get a whipped texture.

Beetroot houmous: Blend 250 g cooked beetroot with a tin of drained cannellini beans, 2 tbsp olive oil, a clove of garlic and a good handful each of mint and dill.

Mint and edamame: Blend 150 g steamed edamame with 2 tbsp reduced-fat Greek yoghurt, the zest and juice of a lemon, 2 handfuls of baby spinach, 2 tbsp olive oil and a handful of mint.

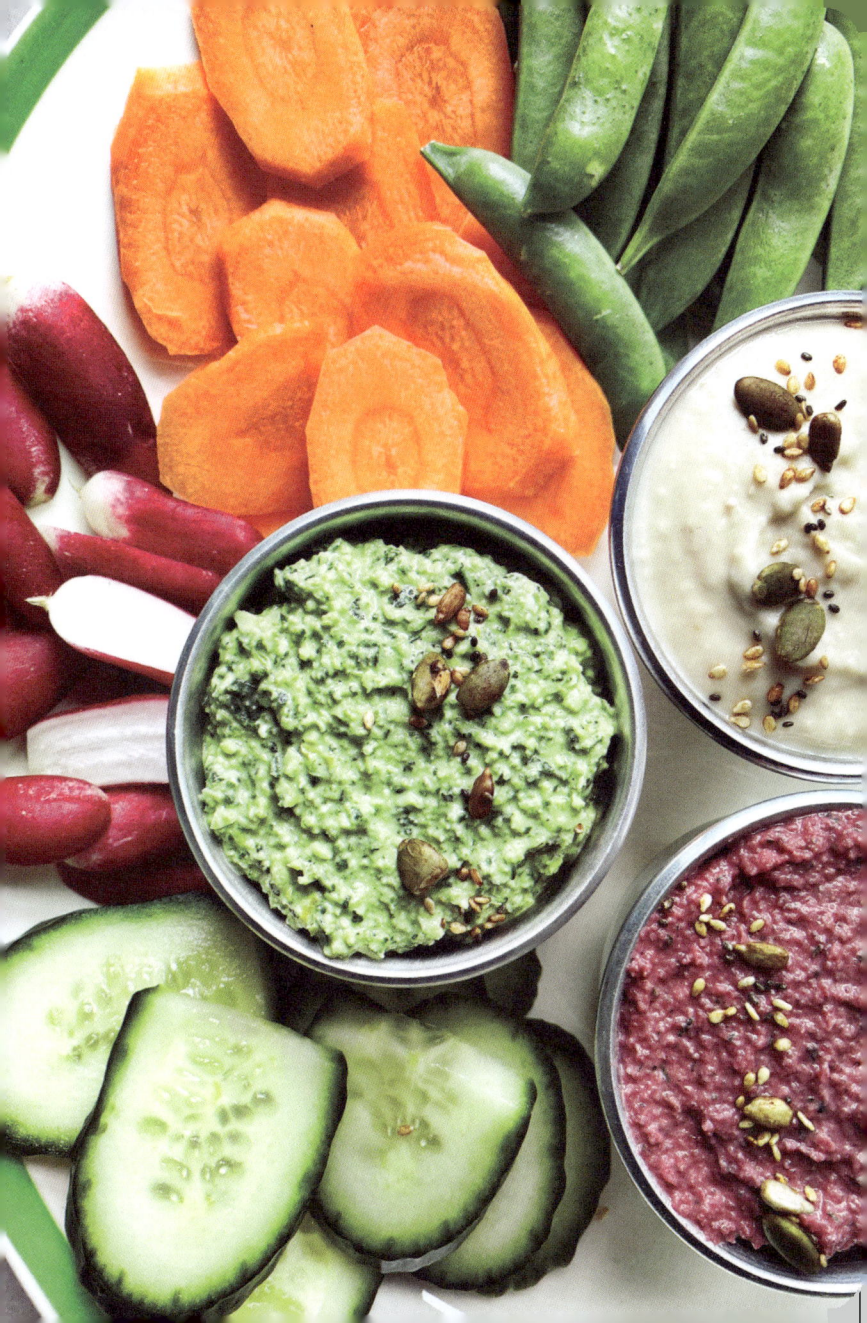

SIMPLE TOMATO SAUCE

Makes one jar | *Ready in 25 mins*

Preheat the oven to 240°C/220°C fan/gas mark 9. Add 12 halved, standard-sized tomatoes to a roasting tin with crushed garlic, dried oregano and black pepper. Drizzle with olive oil and roast for 20 minutes. Blend, then serve with pasta or on little frying pan pizzas (below).

FRYING PAN PIZZAS

Makes two | *Ready in 15 mins*

Mix 250 g self-raising flour, 150 ml water and a pinch of salt. Bring together then knead for 2 minutes. Divide into two and roll into rounds 3 mm thick. Heat your grill.

Meanwhile, drizzle a little olive oil in a small frying pan (that will fit under your grill) and heat the pan on the hob on high. Put the first pizza base into the pan, crisping for about 5 minutes until taking on some colour (use a spatula to check). Top with tomato sauce, grated cheese and halved cherry tomatoes and finish under the grill while still in the pan. Repeat for the second pizza. Top with basil.

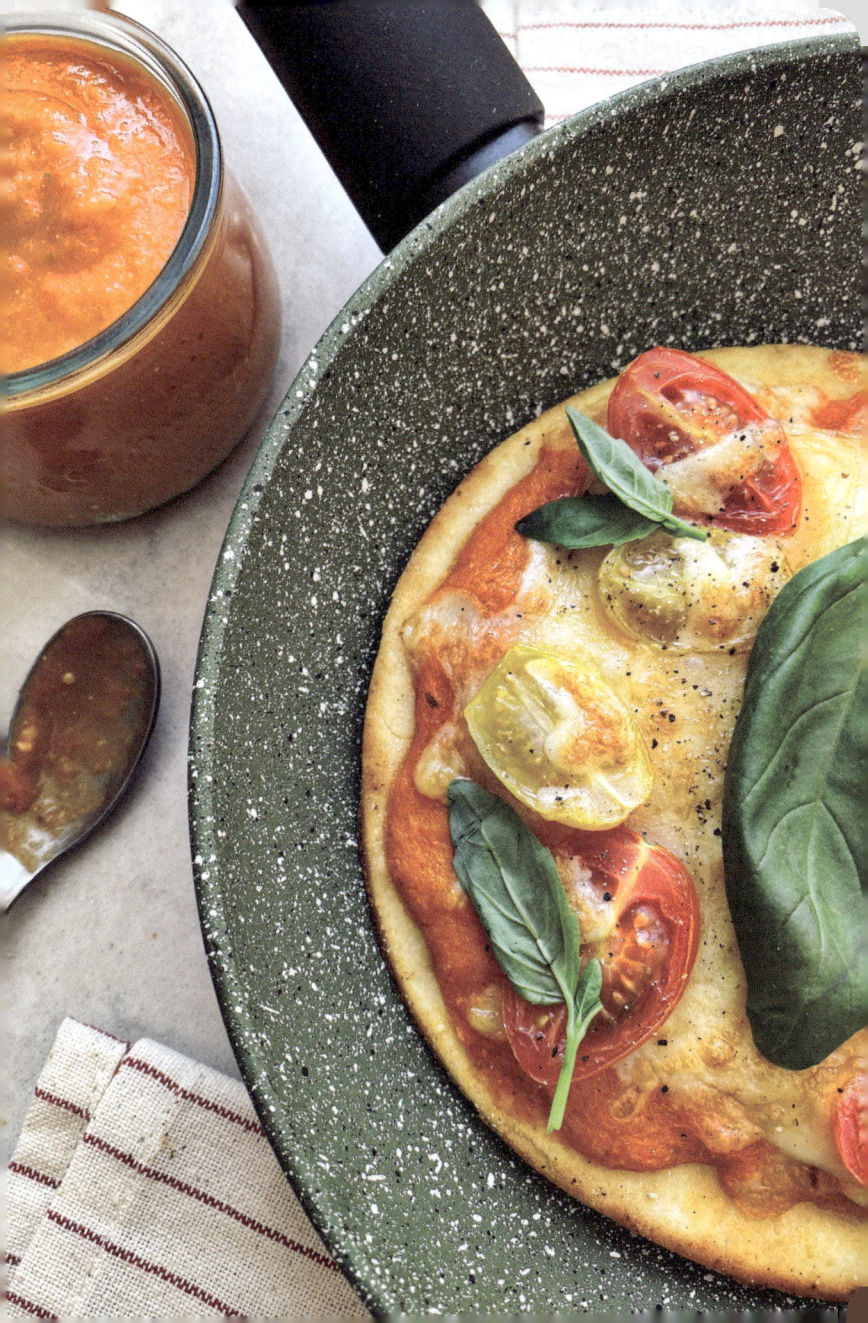

3 PLANT-BASED PASTA SAUCES

All serve two | *All ready in 15–20 mins*

Blend 4 packs of cooked beetroot with 6 tbsp semi-skimmed milk and 2 tbsp olive oil. Stir into cooked tortellini and top with crumbled feta, chopped walnuts and torn basil.

Crumble halloumi into a dry frying pan and cook for a few minutes until crisp. Pop to one side and sauté crushed garlic in the pan with a drizzle of olive oil then add 120 g baby spinach and cook for a minute until wilted. Add to a blender with a good handful each of basil, flat-leaf parsley, pine nuts and grated Parmesan. Blend with 1 tbsp olive oil and stir into cooked ditalini pasta topped with the halloumi crumbs.

Steam 150 g cauliflower until soft with a clove of garlic. Blend with 6 tbsp semi-skimmed milk and 2 tbsp olive oil. Mix into cooked spaghetti, topping with chopped flat-leaf parsley, rocket, grated Parmesan, chopped roasted hazelnuts and black pepper.

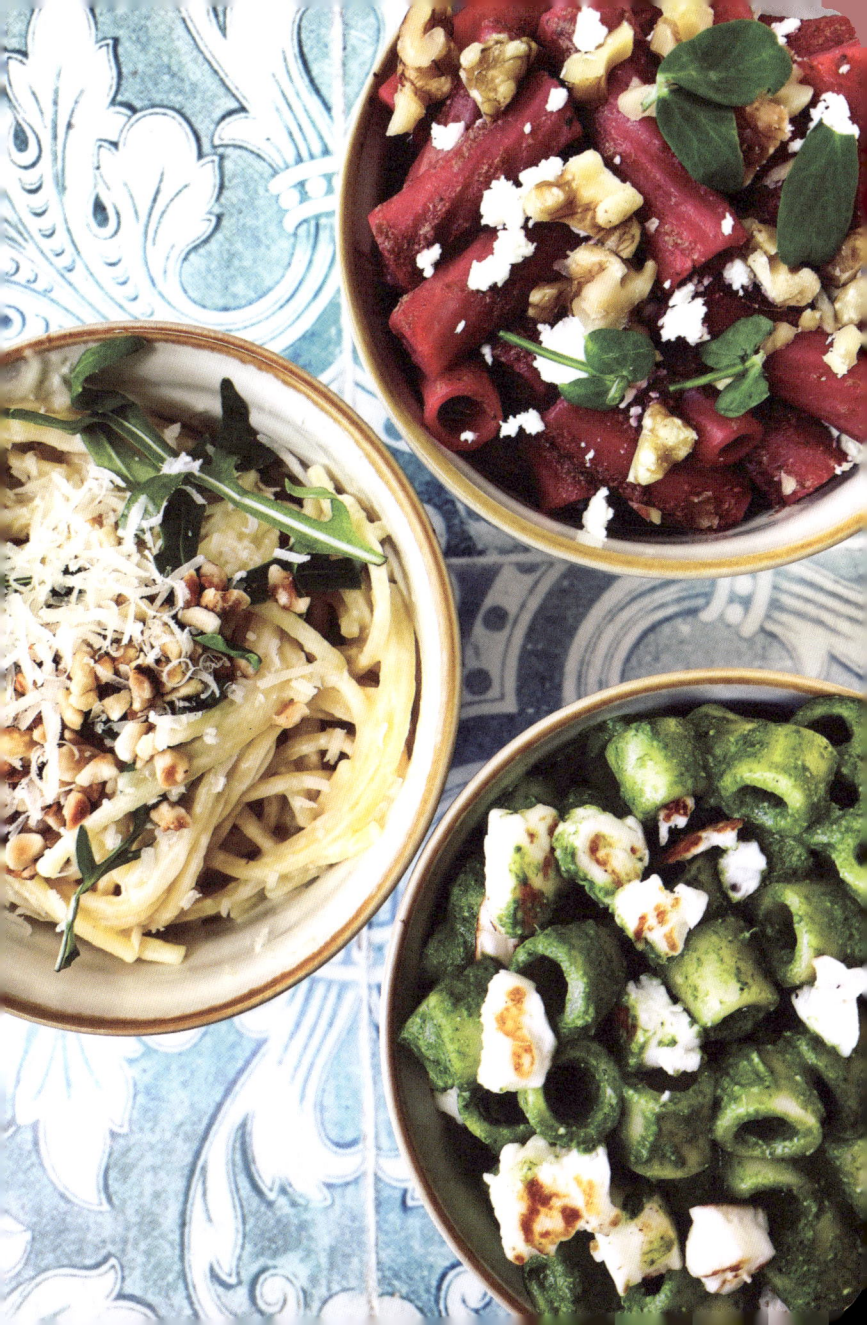

3 SIMPLE MARINADES FOR PROTEIN

Cover chunks of skinless chicken breast or firm tofu in your choice of marinade and refrigerate for at least 30 minutes to 1 hour before cooking (or marinate overnight if you want to get ahead). Marinades make enough for one pack of firm tofu or two large chicken breasts.

All serve two | *All ready in 5 mins + marinating and cooking*

Tikka: Mix the juice of a lemon with 3 tbsp reduced-fat Greek yoghurt, 1 tbsp curry powder, a crushed clove of garlic and grated fresh ginger. (Pictured.)

Teriyaki: Mix 3 tbsp mirin with 2 tbsp reduced-salt soy sauce and 1 tsp honey.

Lemon and herb: Mix the zest and juice of a lemon with 3 tbsp olive oil, a crushed clove of garlic and 2 tsp dried oregano.

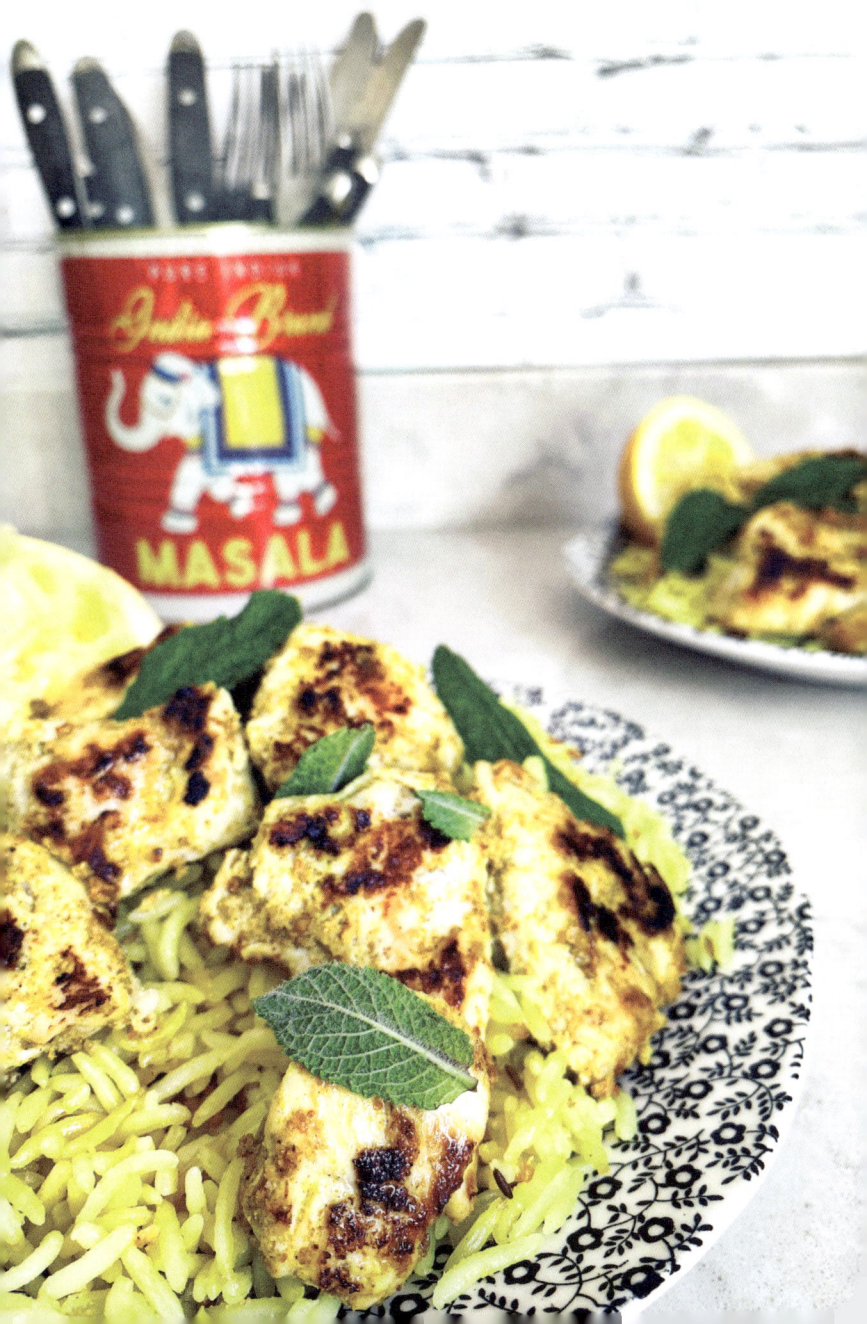

3 IDEAS FOR PULSES AND BEANS

All serve two | *All ready in 20 mins*

Black bean chilli: Soften diced onion, crushed garlic and diced green pepper in olive oil with 1 tsp cumin and 1 tsp chilli powder. Add a drained tin of black beans, a tin of tomatoes and a quarter of a tin of water. Simmer for 15 minutes then serve with chopped avocado and coriander, plus reduced-fat Greek yoghurt. (Pictured.)

Chickpea curry: Soften diced onion in sunflower oil, add crushed garlic and a pinch of dried chilli, fresh grated ginger and 3 tsp curry powder. Stir in a tin of tomatoes, half a tin of water and a drained tin of chickpeas. Simmer for 15 minutes then scatter with chopped coriander and mint. (Pictured.)

Cannellini bean risotto: Heat a 700 g jar of cannellini beans with the stock from the jar. Blend a clove of garlic, a bunch of basil and 3 tbsp olive oil. Once the stock is reduced, take off the heat, grate in Parmesan, like you would a risotto, and stir in the pesto.

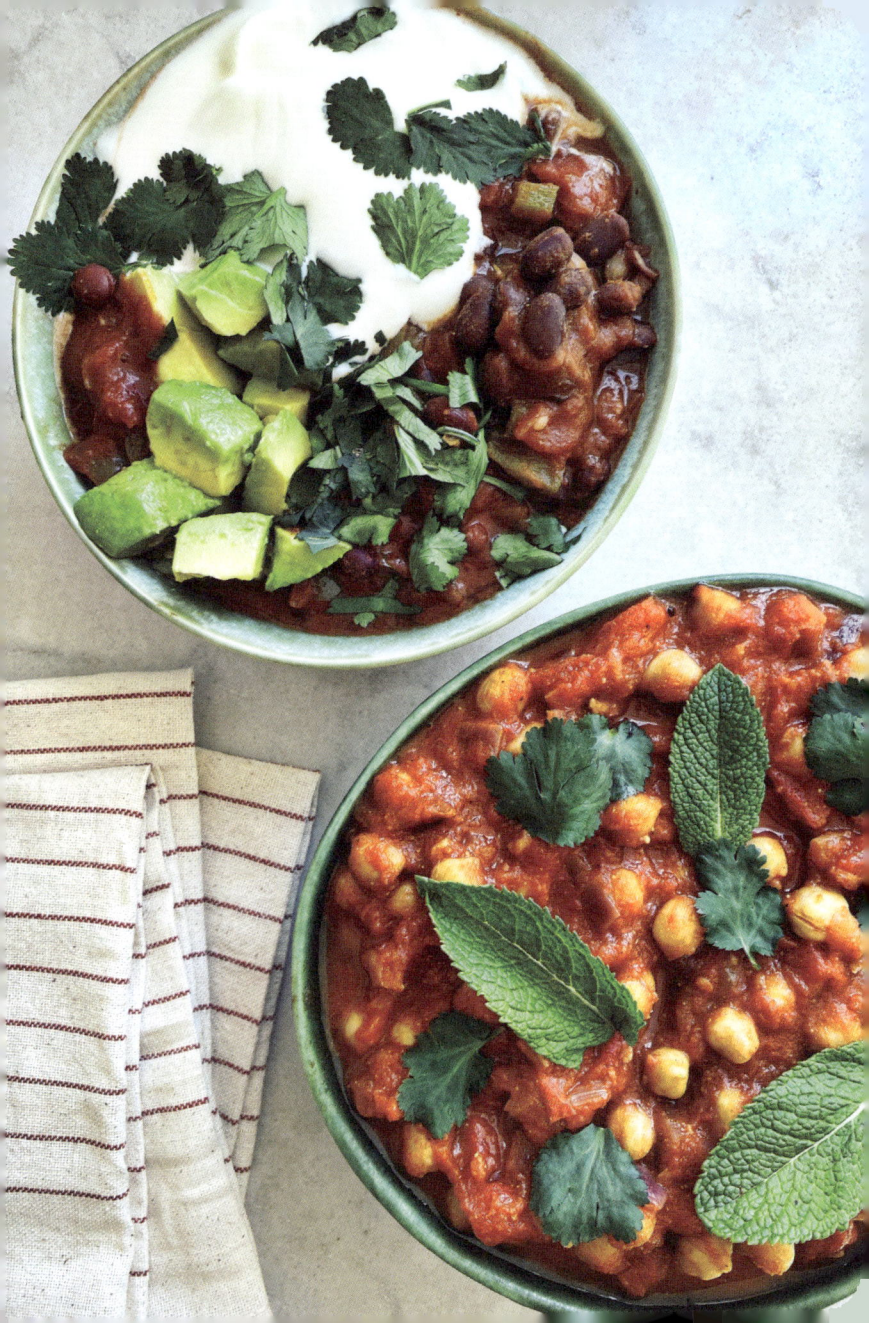

2 SIMPLE STIR-FRIES

Both serve two | *Both ready in 10 mins*

Veggie fried rice: Drizzle a wok with sesame oil and stir-fry a sweet potato cut into 1 cm cubes for 5 minutes with ½ tsp Chinese 5-spice powder, crushed garlic and grated fresh ginger. Add sliced spring onion and a bowl of leftover cold brown rice. Stir-fry for 3 minutes. Mix 1 tbsp reduced-salt soy sauce, 1 tbsp rice vinegar and 1 tsp sriracha. Add to the wok with a handful of frozen edamame and stir-fry for one more minute until piping hot.

Prawn and veggie rice noodles: Cook 2 nests of flat rice noodles according to pack instructions then rinse under cold water. Heat a little sesame oil in a wok, add a handful each of fresh or frozen prawns, finely sliced red or spring onion, bite-sized pieces of broccoli, plus crushed garlic. Stir-fry for 2 minutes. Tip in the noodles with the juice of a lime, 1 tbsp fish sauce and a grated carrot. Toss together for another minute and serve scattered with crushed peanuts, coriander and chilli flakes.

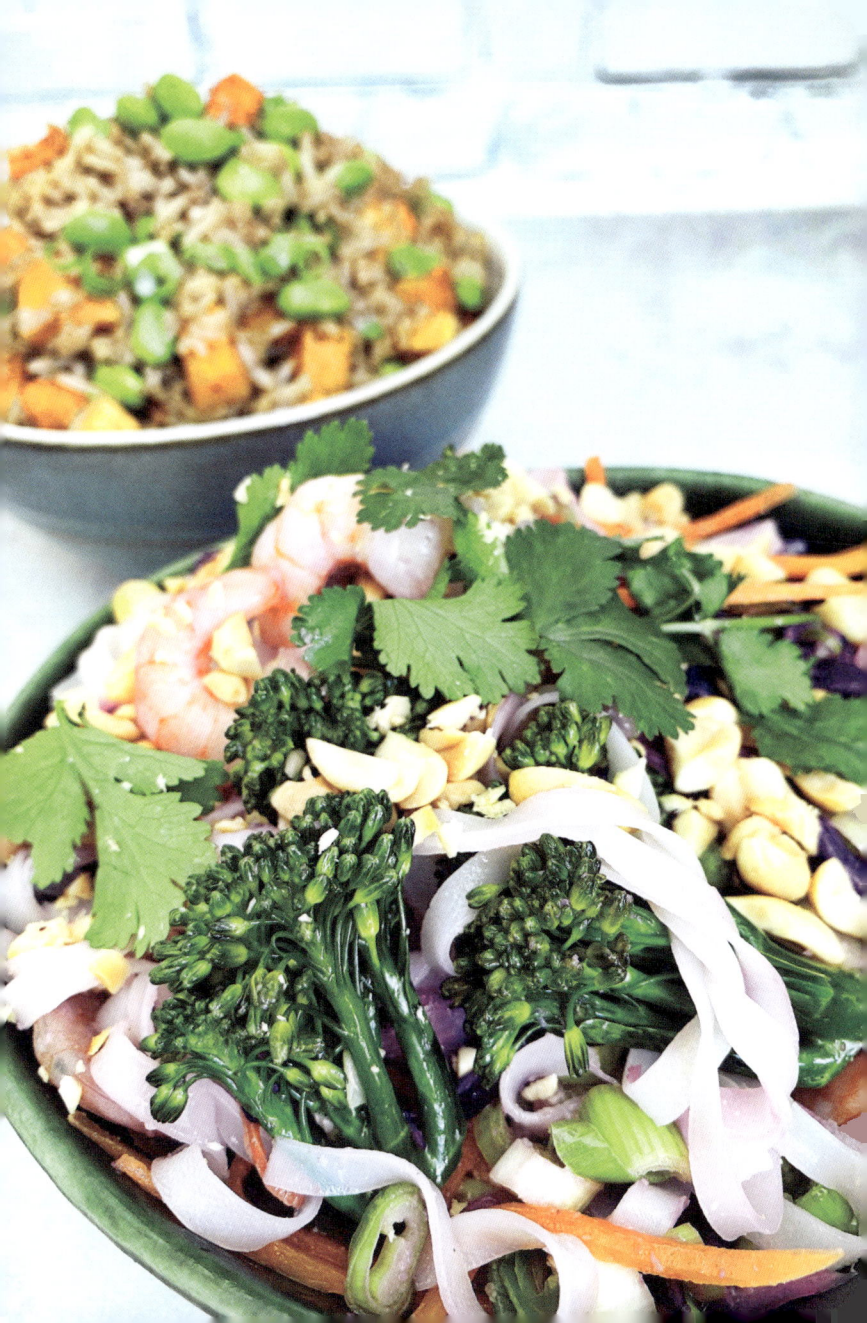

TACOS TWO WAYS

Both serve two | *Both ready in 15 mins + marinating*

Chicken: Mix together the juice and zest of a lime, 2 tbsp olive oil plus 1 tsp each of cumin, paprika and garlic powder. Use to marinate 2 chicken breasts cut into strips (at least 30 minutes to 1 hour). Cook on a griddle pan or barbecue until cooked through.

Veggie: Soften sliced red onion in a drizzle of olive oil with ½ tsp each of cumin, paprika and garlic powder. Add a peeled sweet potato cut into 1-cm cubes and cook for 5 minutes or until soft and browned. Add 2 handfuls of sliced brown mushrooms and cook with everything else until crisp.

TOPPINGS

Take three bowls and add mashed avocado to one, finely diced tomato to the second and shredded green or white cabbage to the third. Mix each with lime juice and chopped coriander. Serve your choice of chicken or veggie filling in soft tacos with the guacamole, tomato salsa, and slaw plus reduced-fat Greek yoghurt to dollop over.

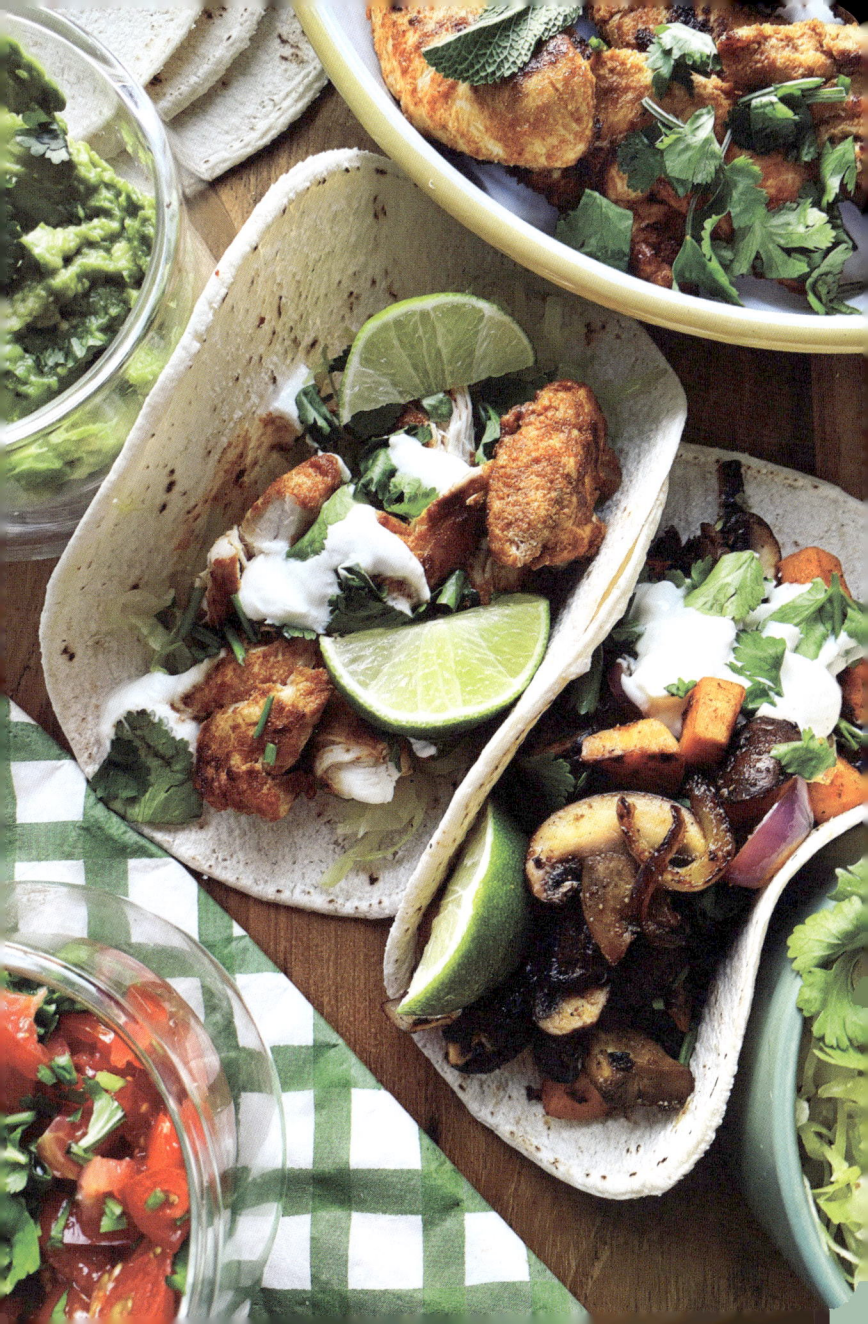

3 MEALS TO MAKE WITH TINNED FISH

All serve two | *All ready in 15 mins or less*

Spaghetti puttanesca: Add chopped anchovies from a tin to a pan with a drizzle of oil from the tin, crushed garlic, a pinch of chilli flakes and 1 tbsp capers. Cook for 2–3 minutes then add 3 diced tomatoes and a handful of chopped black olives. Toss through spaghetti with chopped flat-leaf parsley and basil. (Pictured.)

Warm niçoise salad: Boil baby potatoes and steam green beans. Meanwhile, make a dressing by combining 2 finely chopped tomatoes with 2 finely chopped anchovies, 1 finely sliced spring onion, the juice of half a lemon and finely shredded basil. Mix the hot potatoes and beans with a drained tin of tuna, spoon over the dressing and serve. (Pictured.)

Crab linguine: Mix a drained tin of crab meat with the zest and juice of a lime, a very finely chopped spring onion, chopped flat-leaf parsley and 1 tbsp extra-virgin olive oil. Stir through cooked linguine and sprinkle with dried chilli flakes.

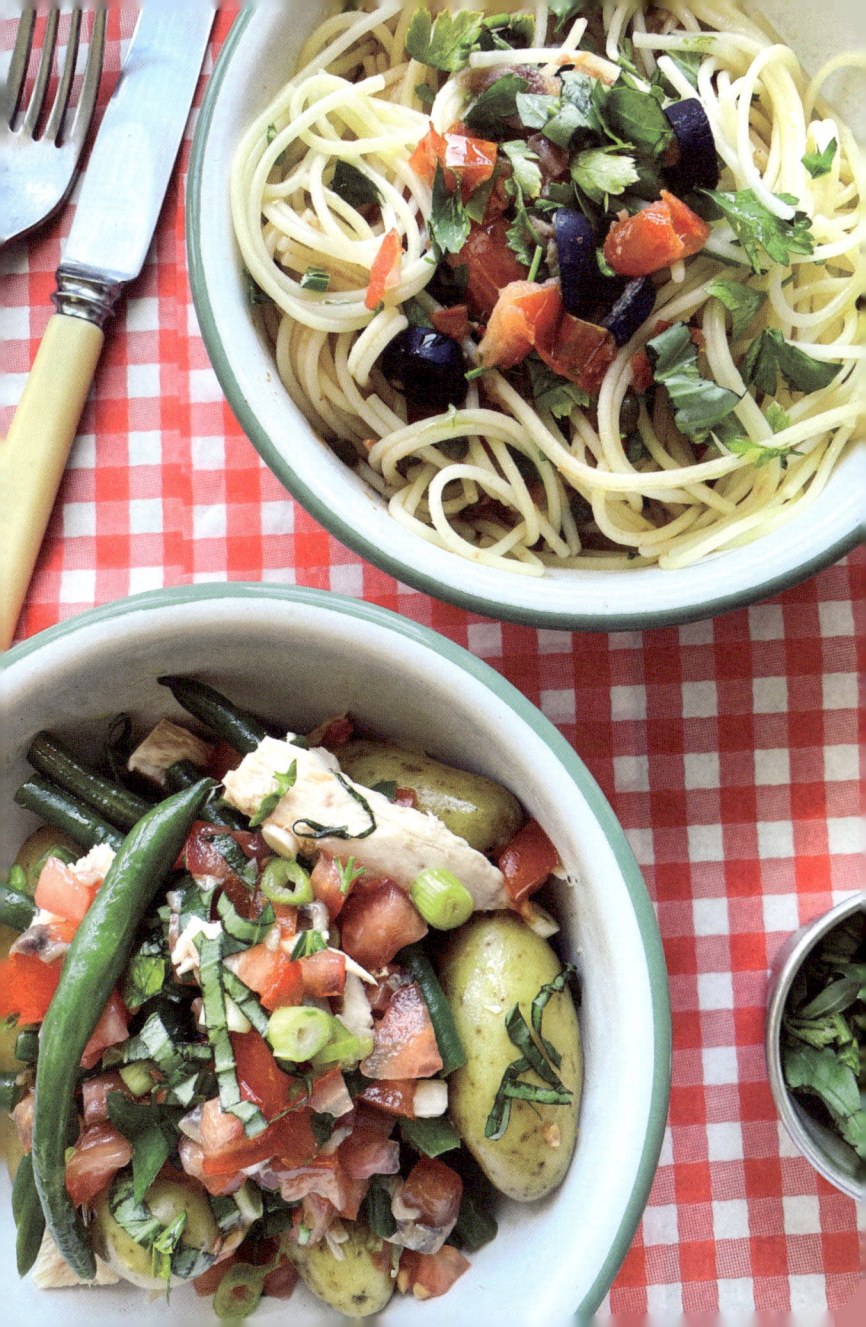

2 MEALS TO MAKE WITH OILY FISH

Both serve four | *Both ready in 20 mins*

Big mack burgers: Soften 2 chopped spring onions in olive oil in a frying pan then pulse in a food processor with 250 g mackerel (skin removed), 100 g spinach, a bunch of coriander and an egg. Remove the blade then stir in 70 g breadcrumbs and the zest of a lemon. Shape into four patties, dust with flour then cook in the frying pan for 8 minutes over a medium heat. Flip and cook for 4 minutes. The burgers will be brown outside and green inside. Serve in buns with salad leaves and beetroot houmous (recipe on p.116). (Pictured.)

Hot smoked-salmon potato salad: Cook 2 handfuls of sliced new potatoes in boiling water. Mix 2 tbsp olive oil, the juice of a lemon, a sliced spring onion and a little chopped flat-leaf parsley. Tear a pack of smoked salmon into pieces and add to a hot frying pan, stirring for 2 minutes until cooked (no need to oil). Drain the potatoes and toss in the dressing whilst warm with the salmon and some mixed leaves.

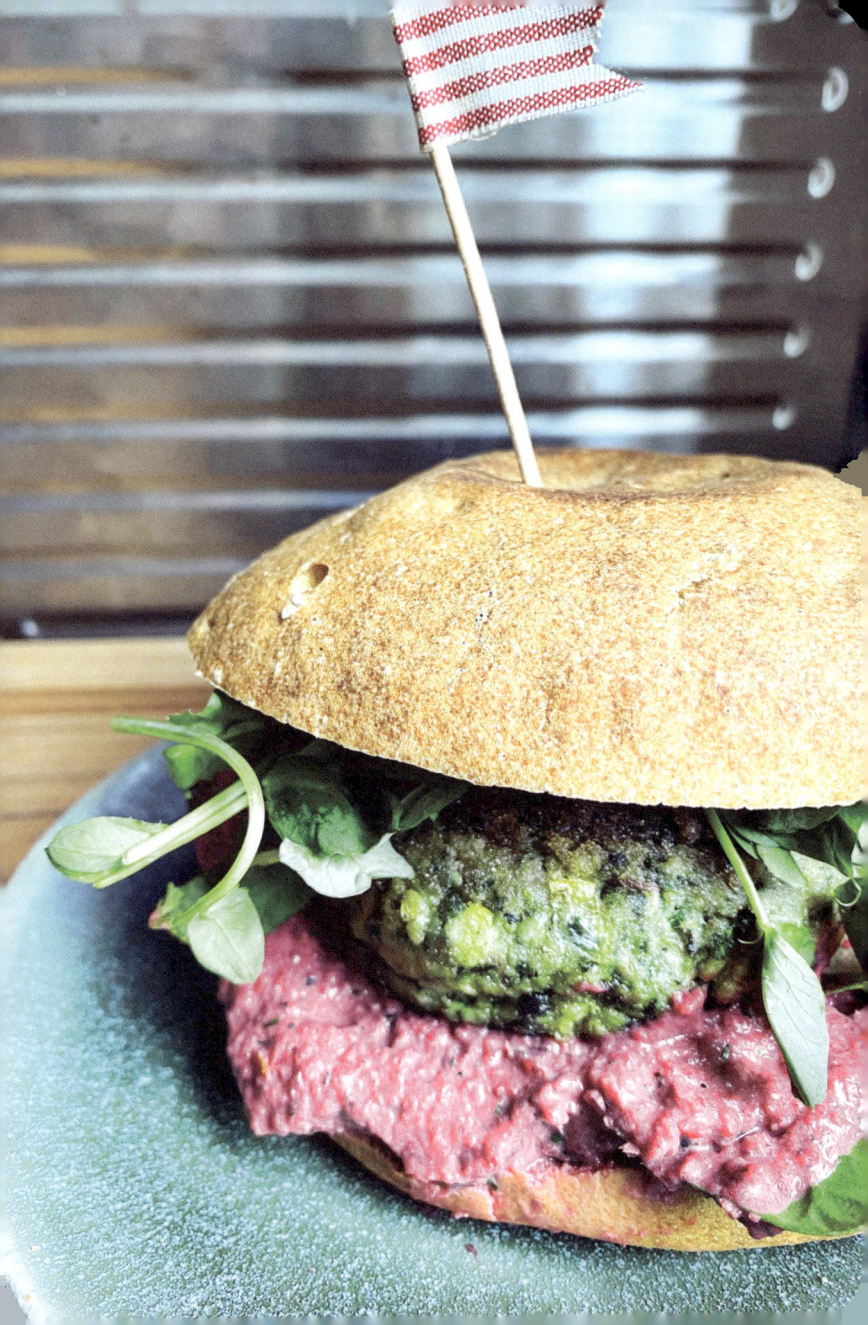

SWEET POTATO FRIES

These moreish fries are roasted in the oven rather than deep-fried. Try them with a salad (see p.94) or big mack burger (see p.132).

Serves two | *Ready in 35 mins*

- 2 sweet potatoes
- dried oregano or cayenne/paprika
- olive oil

Preheat the oven to 200°C/180°C fan/gas mark 6 and line two large baking sheets with baking parchment. Cut the sweet potatoes into 3–5-mm thick strips. Add to a bowl and sprinkle with either dried oregano or a good pinch of cayenne/paprika and a drizzle of olive oil and mix well. Spread out in a single layer on the prepped trays. Cook in the oven for 30–40 minutes, turning halfway through and checking regularly until they're crispy.

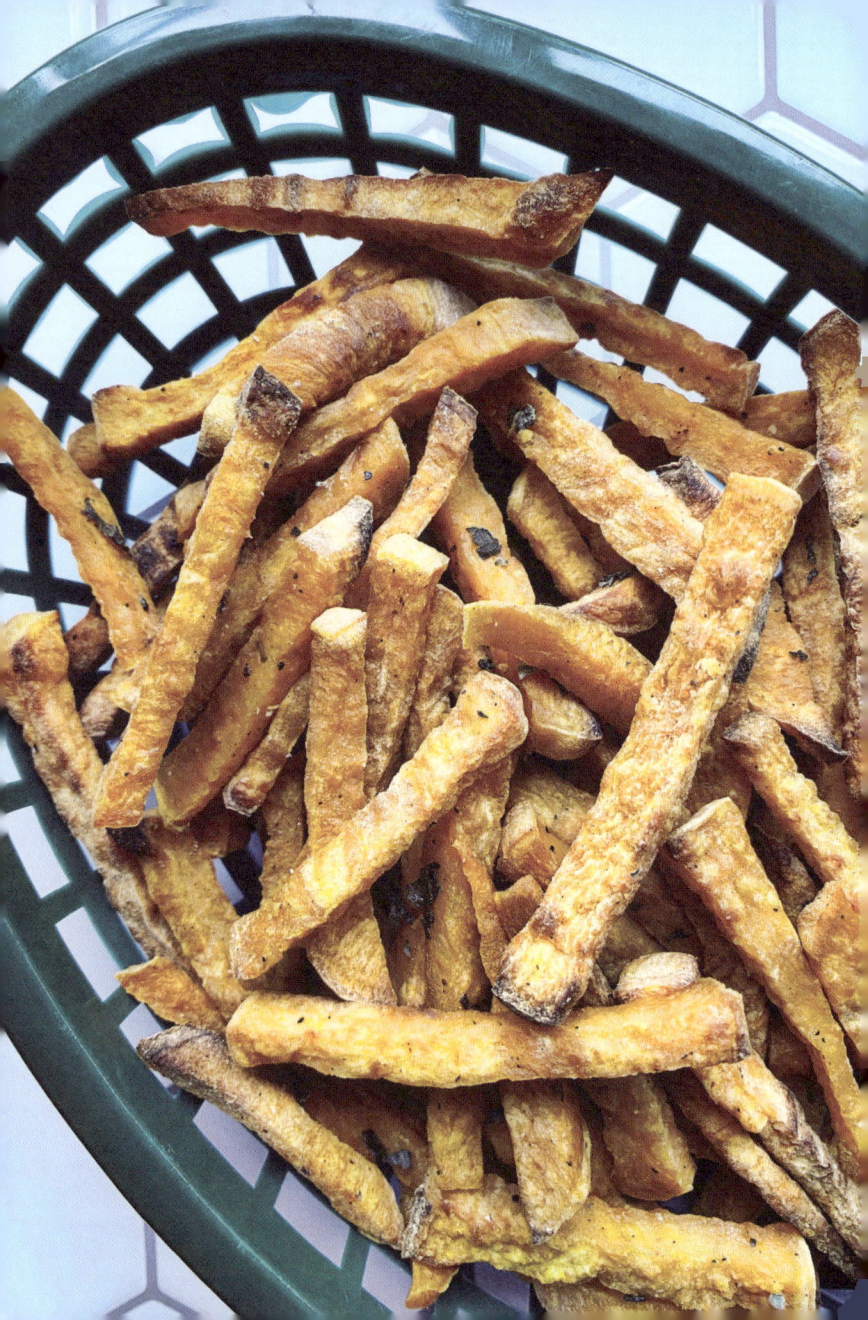

3 MEALS USING MISO

All serve two | *All ready in 45 mins or less*

Japanese chicken salad: Mix shredded cooked chicken and cooked edamame with julienned carrot, celery and cucumber (use a speed peeler). Mix 1 tsp miso, the juice of a lime, grated ginger, 1 tsp sesame oil and 2 tsp hot water. Pour over the salad and scatter with coriander, mint and crunchy seed mix (see p.114). (Pictured.)

Miso aubergine: Preheat the oven to 200°C/180°C fan/gas mark 6. Slice an aubergine lengthways and score a criss-cross pattern in each half. Mix 1 tbsp miso with ½ tbsp sesame oil, ½ tbsp rice vinegar, 1 tsp honey and ½ tbsp hot water and brush over the aubergine. Cook for 35–40 minutes, scatter with coriander and serve with brown rice.

Miso salmon soup: Add 750 ml reduced-salt stock to a pan with 2 handfuls of jasmine rice. Simmer for 12 minutes, adding in the last couple of minutes 1 tbsp miso, 1 tbsp mirin, 1 tbsp reduced-salt soy sauce, grated carrot, sugar snap peas and torn-up smoked salmon. Scatter with coriander.

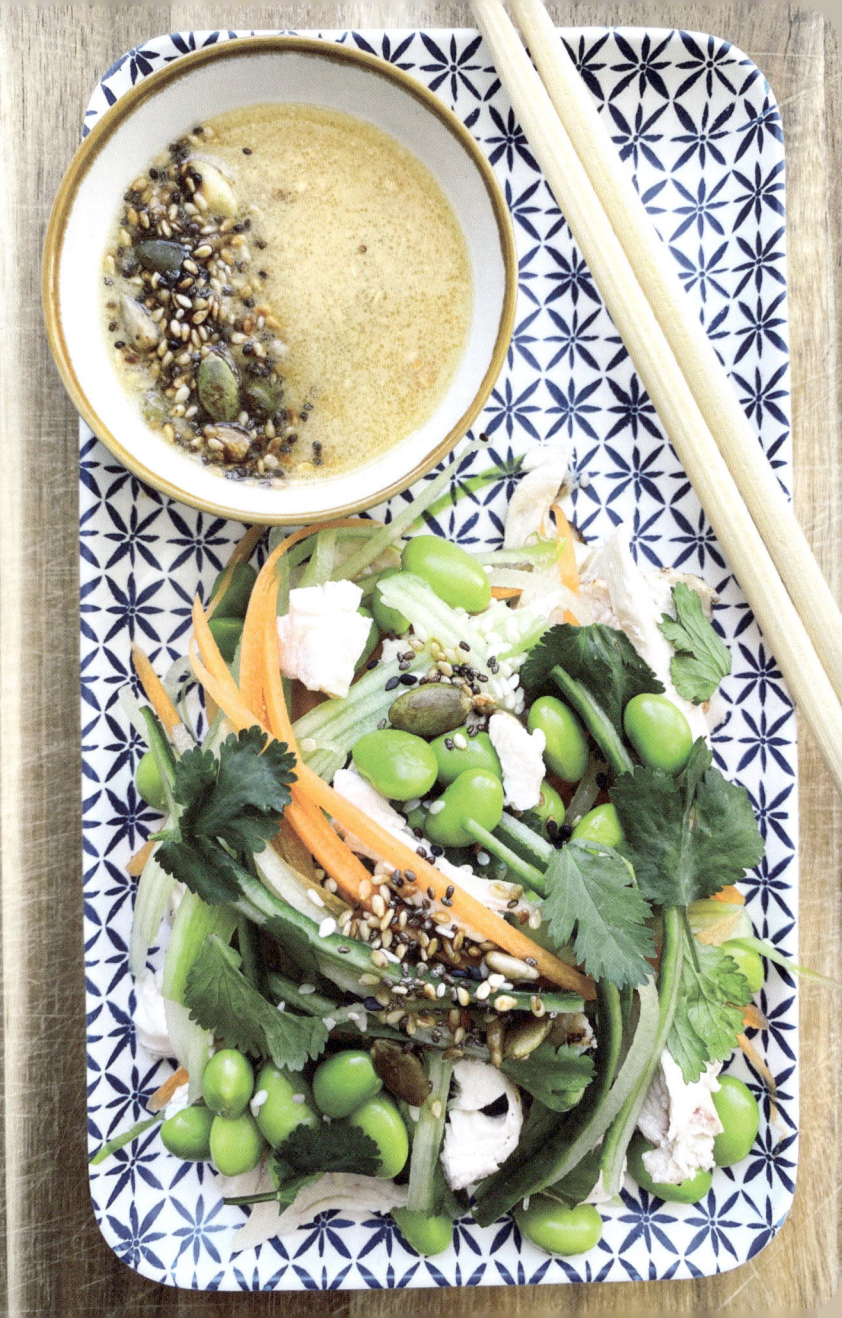

NO-COOK BITE-SIZED SNACKS

ENERGY BALLS
Makes 24 | Ready in 10 mins

Destone 25 Medjool dates then blend in a food processor with 50 g oats, 2 tsp vanilla extract and 4 tbsp cocoa powder. Stop blending when the mixture starts to come away from the sides – this will take a few minutes. Roll the mix into balls with your hands. You can optionally coat these in hazelnuts: just pour a handful of toasted chopped hazelnuts onto a plate and roll the balls in the nuts (do this step as soon as you make them). Store in a jar in the fridge for up to a week.

TRAIL MIX
Makes one 500-ml jar | Ready in 5 mins

Mix together a good handful of dark chocolate chips with a little chopped crystallized ginger. Add a good handful each of toasted, then roughly chopped, cashew nuts, flaked almonds, pumpkin seeds and dried cranberries. Store in a jar for up to a month.

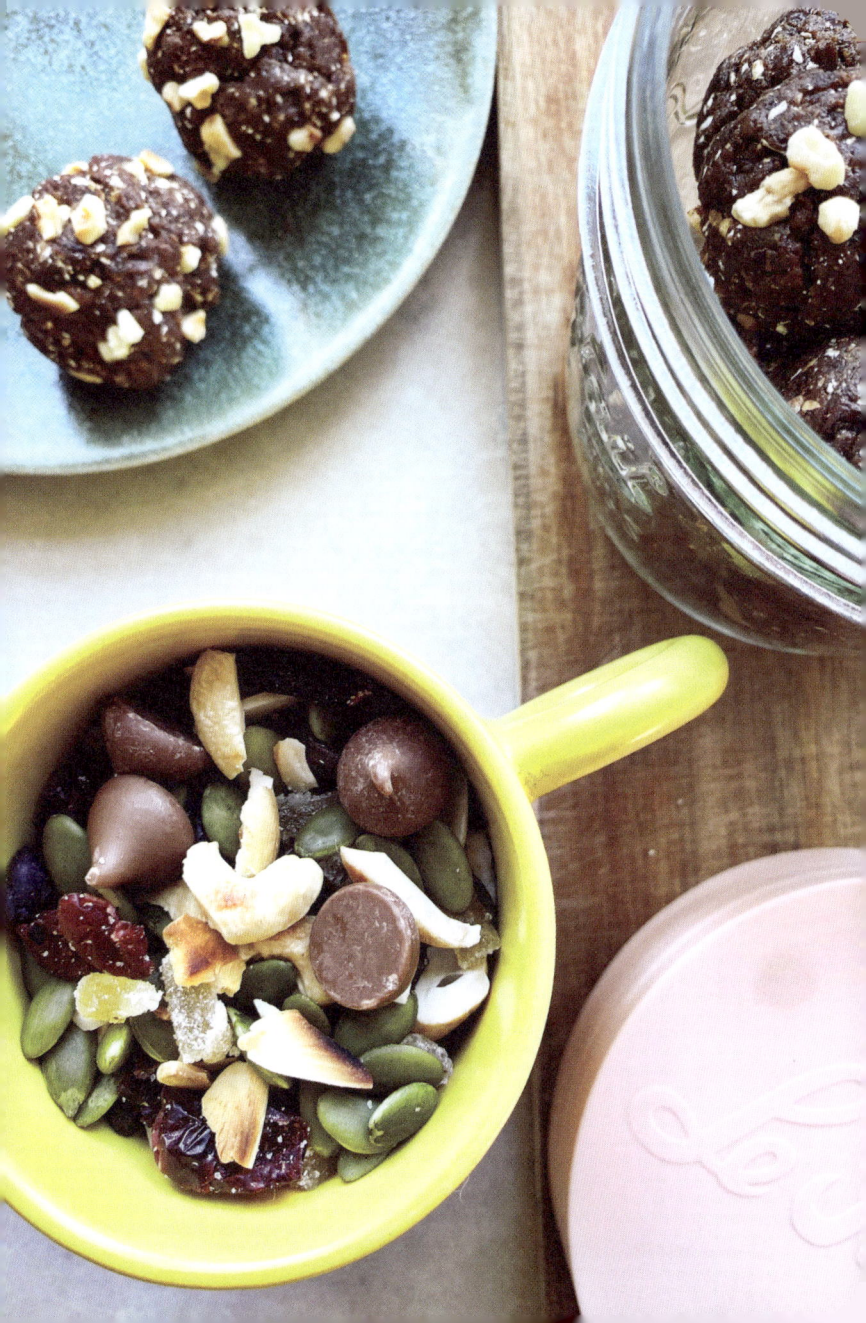

EASY-PREP BANANA BREAD

You don't need weighing scales to make this delicious and reduced-sugar banana bread – everything is easily measured with a spoon. The loaf contains oats, too, for added wholegrains.

Makes one loaf | *Ready in 1 hr + cooling*

- 12 tbsp oats
- 5 tbsp self-raising flour
- 1 tsp bicarbonate of soda
- 3 tbsp chopped pecans
- 3 very ripe bananas + 1 extra for the top
- 5 tbsp sunflower oil
- 3 tbsp honey

Preheat the oven to 200°C/180°C fan/gas mark 6 and grease and line a 450 g (1 lb) loaf tin. Blend the oats until fine like flour. Add to a bowl with the self-raising flour, bicarbonate of soda and pecans. Mash three of the bananas then mix with the sunflower oil and honey. Fold into the flour mix then add to the tin. Slice the extra banana in half lengthways and gently place into the top of the batter. Bake for 40 minutes, covering with foil if it is browning too much. Leave to cool completely in the tin before removing.

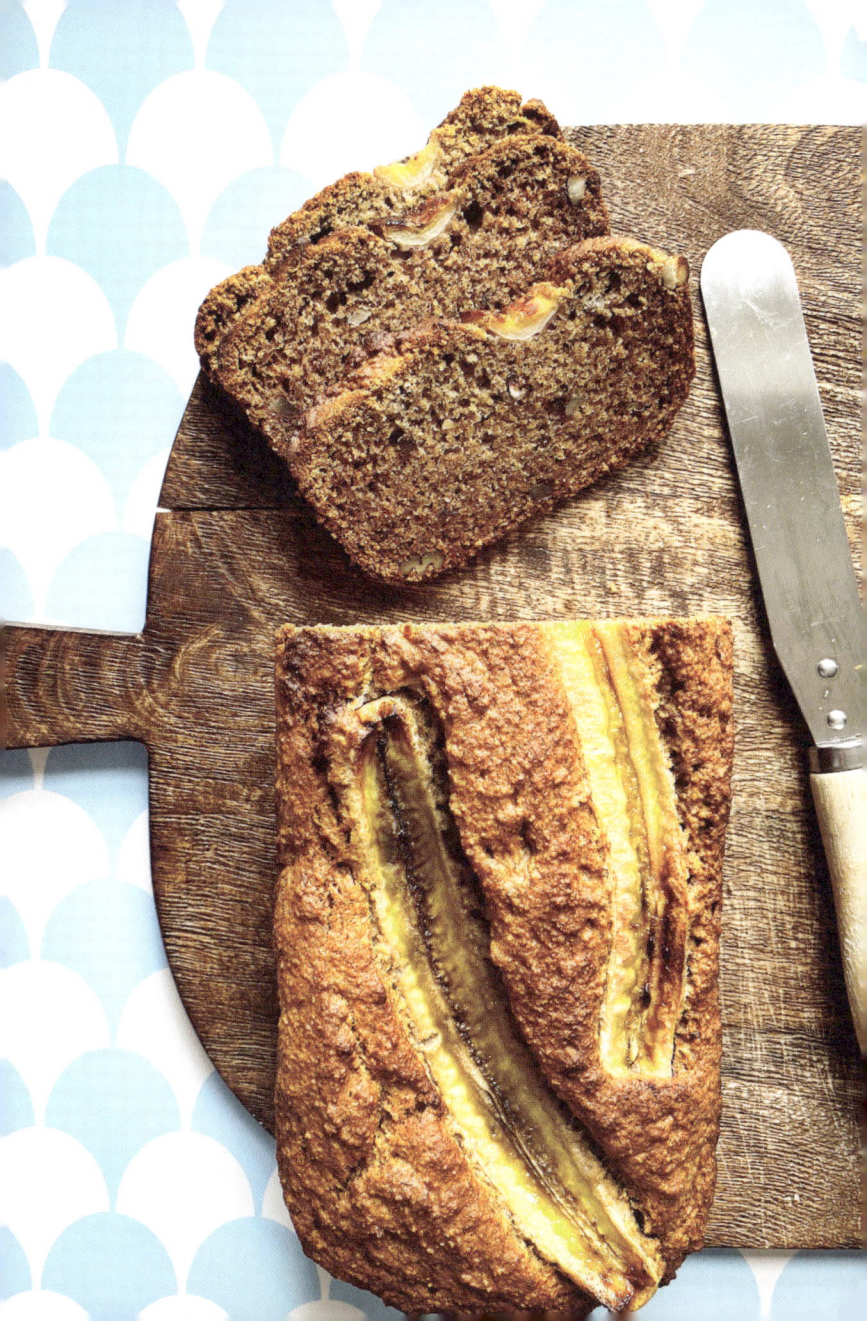

RASPBERRY AND PISTACHIO BROWNIE BARS

These fudgy brownies have a secret ingredient: sweet potato. The recipe makes little bars and is simple to whip up in a food processor.

Makes eight | *Ready in 40 mins*

- 250 g sweet potato
- 4 tbsp honey
- 3½ tbsp peanut butter
- 1 tbsp sunflower oil
- 3 tbsp cocoa powder
- 5 tbsp oats
- 1 tsp baking powder
- 1 tsp vanilla extract

TOPPINGS

- 1 handful each of chopped pistachios, dark chocolate chips and frozen raspberries

Preheat the oven to 180°C/160°C fan/gas mark 4 and line an 18 x 24-cm baking sheet with baking parchment. Peel the sweet potato, cut into small cubes and steam for 10 minutes. Blend until smooth in a food processer. Add the rest of the ingredients to the processor and blend again. Transfer to the baking sheet and spread evenly. Sprinkle over the toppings, pressing everything down with the back of a spoon. Bake for 25 minutes then cool completely in the tin before slicing.

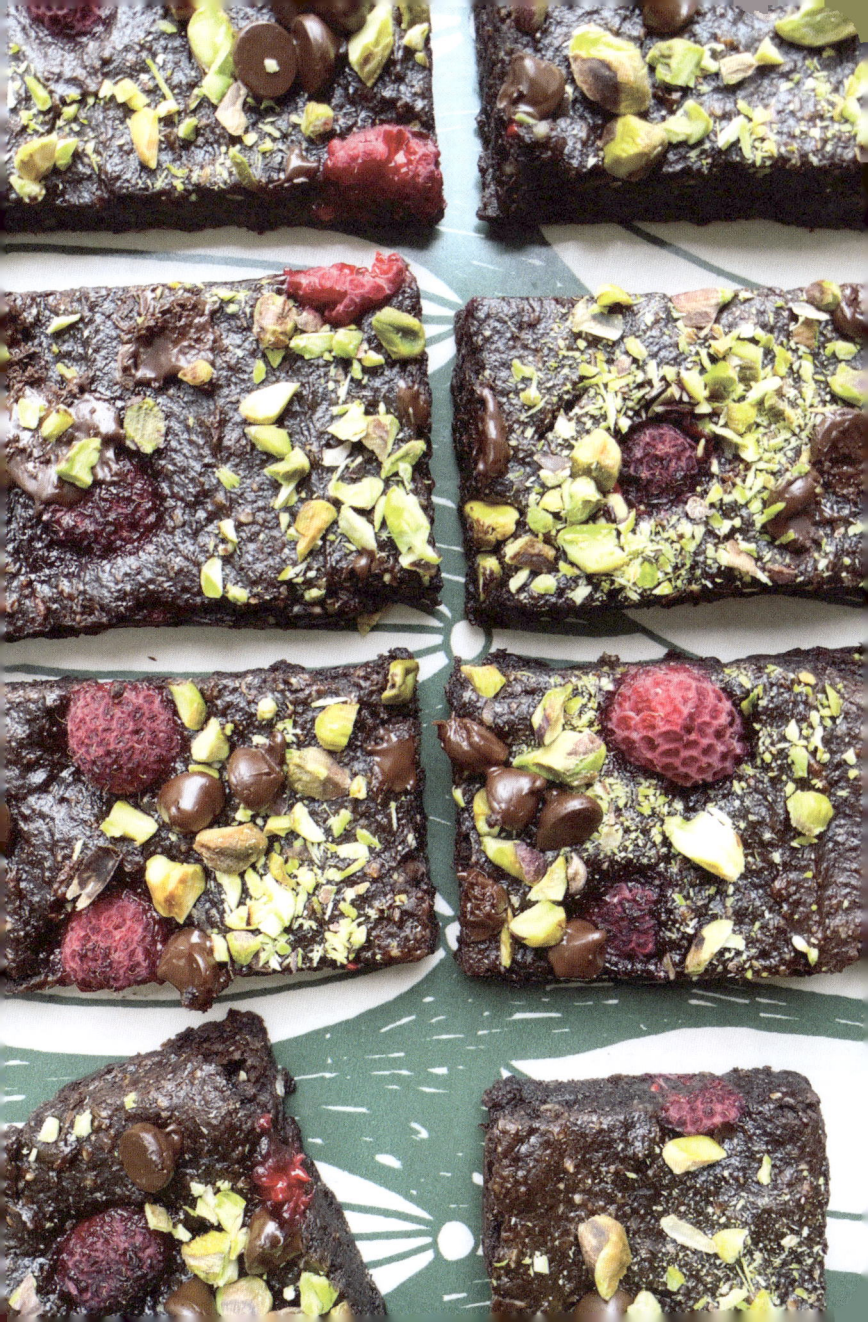

CHOCOLATE CHIP COOKIES

These cookies are made with chickpeas and peanut butter to boost the protein, whilst keeping them lovely and soft. They contain less sugar than standard cookies but are just as moreish. Best made with peanut butter containing no added oil.

Makes 12 | *Ready in 20 mins*

- 1 tin of chickpeas
- 220 g smooth peanut butter
- 2 tbsp honey
- 1 tsp vanilla extract
- 1 tsp bicarbonate of soda
- 80 g dark chocolate chips

Preheat the oven to 180°C/160°C fan/gas mark 4 and line a large baking sheet with parchment. Drain the chickpeas and add to a food processor with the peanut butter, honey, vanilla extract and bicarbonate of soda. Whizz until the mixture starts to come away from the sides then remove the blade and stir in the chocolate chips. Roll 12 balls of dough by hand, adding to the tray then flattening slightly with the back of a spoon. Bake for 12 minutes, cool on the tray for 5 minutes, then remove to a wire rack to cool completely.

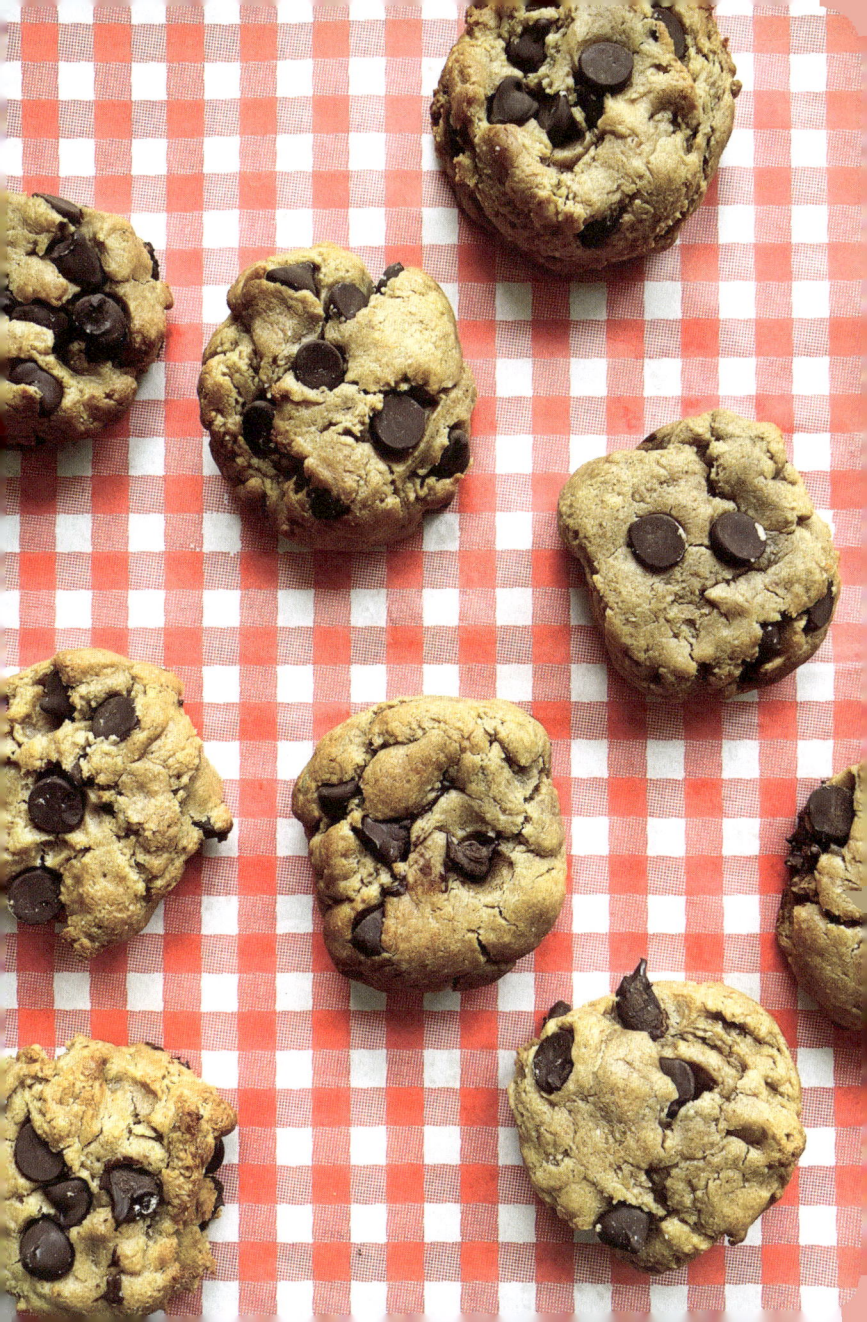

PEANUT BUTTER CUPS

Everybody's favourite combination with only four ingredients. Keep a jar on standby in the fridge to satisfy chocolate cravings.

Makes eight | Ready in 15 mins + freezing

- 200 g milk or dark chocolate chips
- 1½ tbsp smooth peanut butter
- ½ tsp honey
- ½ tsp vanilla extract

Melt the chocolate chips. Use a teaspoon to add a little to the bottom of 8 holes in a silicone mini cupcake mould. Pop in the freezer to set (about 5 minutes). Meanwhile, mix together the peanut butter, honey and vanilla extract. Once set, remove the silicone mould from the freezer and add a dollop of the peanut mix to the centre of each chocolate disc, leaving a little space around the edges. Spoon the remaining chocolate into the 8 moulds, ensuring it fills to the edges. Level off the top with a teaspoon and return to the freezer to set for 15 minutes then pop out of the cases. Store in the fridge until ready to eat.

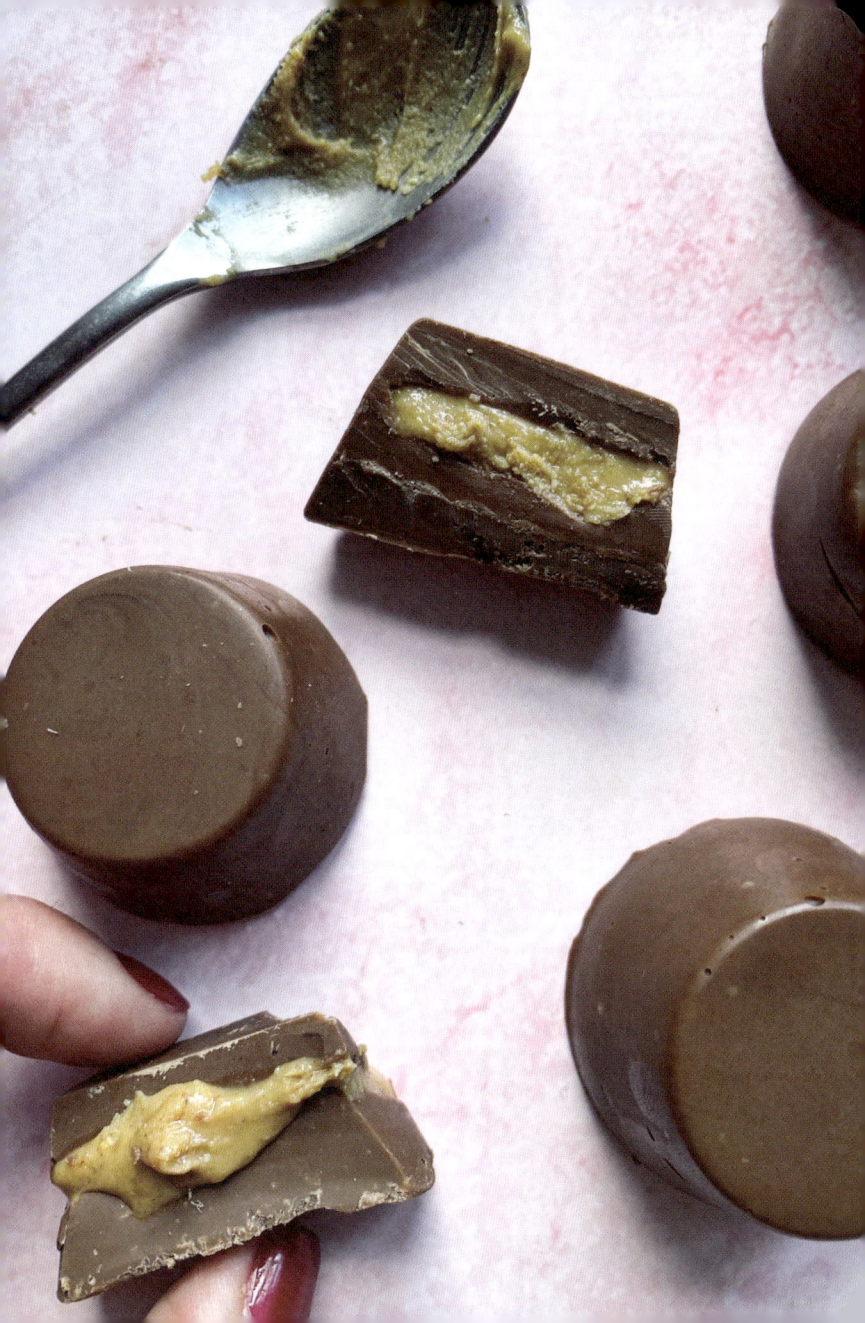

STRAWBERRIES AND CREAM FROZEN YOGHURT

There are only four ingredients in this dessert. It's sweetened with strawberries plus a little honey.

Makes one tub | *Ready in 10 mins + freezing*

- 300 g strawberries, hulled
- 300 ml crème fraîche
- 500-g tub Greek yoghurt
- 4 tsp honey

Roughly chop 150 g of the strawberries. Add the remaining strawberries to a food processor and blend with the crème fraiche, yoghurt and honey until combined. Mix in the chopped strawberries then spoon into a large loaf tin or other suitable container, top with baking parchment and freeze overnight.

TOP TIPS

For creamier yoghurt, remove from the freezer once or twice during initial freezing and whisk with a fork. This helps prevent ice crystals forming. Take out of the freezer about 30 minutes before you want to serve it. Can be stored in the freezer for up to a month.

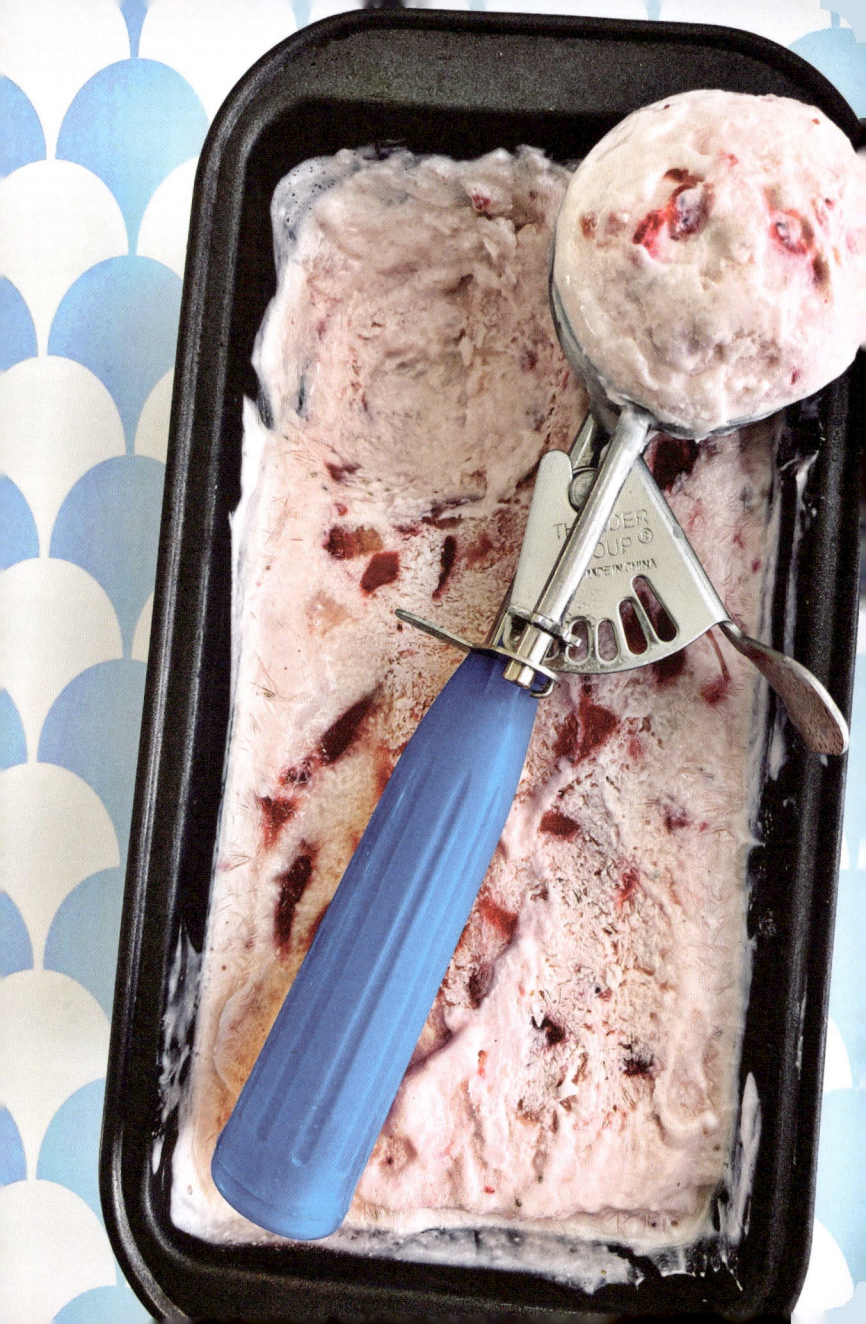

		Dairy-free	Nut-free	Gluten-free
p.90	5 ways to top a baked potato	A	☑	☑
p.92	3 balanced sandwiches	A	☑	A
p.94	3 superfood salads	A		☑
p.96	3 salad dressings	☑	☑	☑
p.98	3 meals to make with avocados	A	A	A
p.100	3 big-batch breakfast cereals	☑		A
p.102	3 ideas for overnight oats	A		A
p.104	3 protein-rich breakfasts	A		A
p.106	Seeded oat bread	A	☑	A
p.108	Green protein waffles			A
p.110	Matcha smoothie	A	☑	A
p.112	2 simple soups	A	☑	A
p.114	Crunchy seed mix	☑	☑	A
p.114	Leek and cannellini bean soup	A	☑	A
p.116	3 easy dips	A	☑	☑
p.118	Simple tomato sauce	A	☑	A
p.118	Frying pan pizzas	A	☑	A
p.120	3 plant-based pasta sauces	A		A
p.122	3 simple marinades for protein	A	☑	A
p.124	3 ideas for pulses and beans	A	☑	☑
p.126	2 simple stir-fries	☑		A
p.128	Tacos two ways	A	☑	A
p.130	3 ideas with tinned fish	☑	☑	A
p.132	2 meals to make with oily fish	☑	☑	A
p.134	Sweet potato fries	☑	☑	☑
p.136	3 meals using miso	☑	☑	A
p.138	No-cook bite-sized snacks	A		A
p.140	Easy-prep banana bread	☑		A
p.142	Raspberry and pistachio brownie bars	A		A
p.144	Chocolate chip cookies	A		A
p.146	Peanut butter cups	A		A
p.148	Frozen yoghurt		☑	☑

A = adapt by using dairy-free or gluten-free alternative – e.g. dairy-free cheese or yoghurt or gluten-free bread, pasta or oats

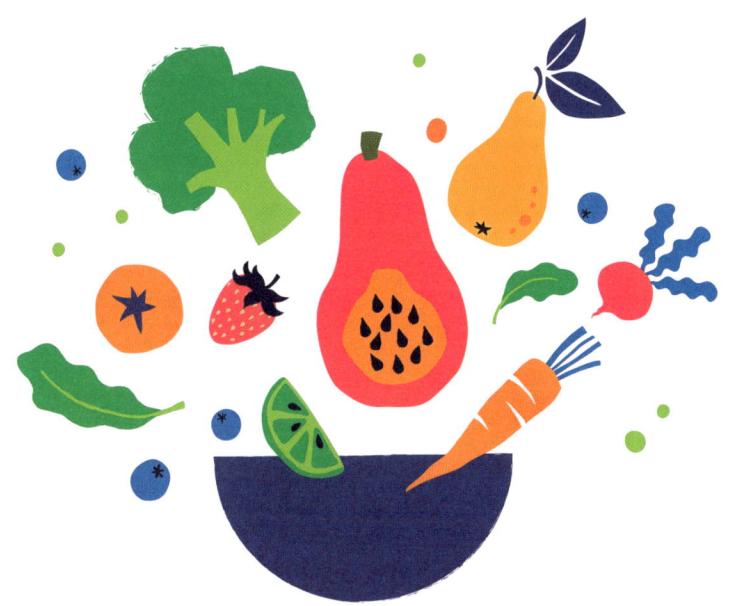

Chapter Four:
WEEKLY MEAL PLANS

This chapter contains three full weekly meal plans for breakfast, lunch, dinner, dessert and snacks. Choose from an easy-prep, speedy or affordable plan or mix-and-match different days from different plans. Each provides you with a balanced set of meals to enjoy throughout the week, and you'll find all the recipes in the Nutrition Hacks chapter (p.64). For tips on making your own meal plans, see p.83.

Easy-prep

To ease daily food prep, you can make many elements of this plan the weekend before the Monday, including the granola, banana and oat breads and energy balls. You can slice the oat bread and freeze it to toast from frozen as you need it. All the lunches can be prepped the night before you eat them, and the tortellini soup base, chickpea curry and chicken marinade can all also be prepped ahead of time.

	MONDAY	**TUESDAY**	**WEDNESDAY**
Breakfast	Granola (p.100) with yoghurt and berries	Overnight granola jar (p.102)	Avocado jar (p.98) with toasted sourdough
Lunch	Chicken and avocado sandwich (p.92) with veggie sticks	Easy dip (p.116) with veggie sticks and oatcakes	Tuna mix (p.90) in a sandwich with slaw (p.90)
Dinner	Tortellini soup (p.112)	Chickpea curry (p.124) with brown rice	Broccoli baked potato (p.90)
Dessert/ Snacks	Banana bread (p.140)	Apple slices with nut butter	Energy balls (p.138)

	THURSDAY	**FRIDAY**	**SATURDAY**	**SUNDAY**
Breakfast	Seeded oat bread (p.106) spread with reduced-fat Greek yoghurt and berries	Granola (p.100) with semi-skimmed milk and sliced banana	Smoked salmon with reduced-fat cream cheese (p.104) on seeded oat bread (p.106)	Scrambled eggs on toasted seeded oat bread (p.106) or breakfast tacos (p.104)
Lunch	Leek and cannellini bean soup with feta and crunchy seed mix (p.114)	Leftover slaw with grated carrot mix, feta and sweetcorn salad (all p.90)	Buddha bowl or another salad (both p.94)	Easy dip (p.116) with veggie sticks and oatcakes
Dinner	Lemon and herb marinated chicken (p.122) with slaw (p.90)	Avocado pesto pasta (p.98) with a cooked salmon fillet	Simple stir-fry (p.126)	Hot smoked-salmon potato salad (p.132)
Dessert/ Snacks	Piece of fruit	Oatcakes with nut butter	Energy balls (p.138)	Banana bread (p.140)

Speedy

Make the muesli, oat bread, trail mix, crunchy seed mix and slaw in advance to ensure you can get food on the table fast when you need it. You can slice the oat bread and freeze it to toast from frozen. Make all the lunches, the overnight oats and marinate the chicken tikka the night before you'll eat them. All dinners are ready in 15 minutes or less.

	MONDAY	**TUESDAY**	**WEDNESDAY**
Breakfast	Muesli (p.100) with semi-skimmed milk and sliced banana	Carrot cake overnight oats (p.102)	Seeded oat bread (p.106) with nut butter and blueberries
Lunch	Coronation chickpea sandwich (p.92) with veggie sticks	Easy dip (p.116) with veggie sticks and oatcakes	Mini mozzarella balls with tomato and basil (p.94) mixed with a tin of lentils or a pouch of brown rice
Dinner	Miso salmon soup (p.136)	Beetroot pasta (p.120) with slaw (p.90)	Avocado pesto pasta (p.98) with a cooked salmon fillet
Dessert/ Snacks	Trail mix (p.138)	Piece of fruit	Crunchy seed mix (p.114)

	THURSDAY	**FRIDAY**	**SATURDAY**	**SUNDAY**
Breakfast	Blueberry and banana overnight oats (p.102)	Muesli (p.100) with semi-skimmed milk and berries	Avocado smoothie bowl (p.98)	Quinoa porridge (p.104) with nut butter, berries and reduced-fat Greek yoghurt
Lunch	Chicken and avocado sandwich (p.92) and slaw (p.90)	Tuna mix (p.90) in sandwich with slaw (p.90)	Easy dip (p.116) with veggie sticks and oatcakes	Halloumi, broccoli and grain salad (p.94)
Dinner	Cheat's pho (p.112)	Chicken tikka, (p.122) with a warmed pouch of brown rice, sliced cucumber, chopped green pepper, mint and a dollop of reduced-fat Greek yoghurt	Prawn and veggie rice noodles (p.126)	Crab linguine (p.130)
Dessert/ Snacks	Piece of fruit	Trail mix (p.138)	Apple slices with nut butter	Crunchy seed mix (p.114)

Affordable

This plan makes good use of economical ingredients including frozen fruit and veg, and tinned fish, beans and lentils. Use leftovers and nutritious staples like oats on different days to make money go further.

	MONDAY	**TUESDAY**	**WEDNESDAY**
Breakfast	Quinoa porridge (p.104) with nut butter, defrosted frozen berries and reduced-fat Greek yoghurt	Reduced-fat Greek yoghurt with defrosted frozen berries and seeds or nuts	Quinoa porridge (p.104) with nut butter, defrosted frozen berries and reduced-fat Greek yoghurt
Lunch	Easy dip (p.116) with veggie sticks and oatcakes	Grated carrot salad (p.90) mixed with drained tinned lentils	Feta and sweetcorn salad (p.90) mixed with a drained tin of mixed beans
Dinner	Baked potato with tuna mix (p.90) and green salad	Black bean chilli (p.124)	Miso salmon soup (p.136)
Dessert/ Snacks	Piece of fresh fruit	Energy balls (p.138)	Apple slices with nut butter

	THURSDAY	**FRIDAY**	**SATURDAY**	**SUNDAY**
Breakfast	Frozen fruit and oat smoothie (p.84)	Seeded oat bread (p.106) with nut butter and defrosted frozen blueberries	Scrambled eggs on toasted seeded oat bread (p.106) with halved cherry tomatoes	Seeded oat bread (p.106) with nut butter and defrosted frozen blueberries
Lunch	Easy dip (p.116) with veggie sticks and oatcakes	Chicken and avocado sandwich (p.92)	Leek and cannellini bean soup with crumbled feta (p.114)	Broccoli baked potato (p.90) – use frozen broccoli
Dinner	Spaghetti puttanesca (p.130)	Sweet potato and mushroom tacos (p.128)	Frying pan pizza (p.118) with slaw (p.90)	Wholewheat pasta with leftover tomato sauce from the pizza + leftover slaw (p.90)
Dessert/Snacks	Piece of fresh fruit	Energy balls (p.138)	Apple slices with nut butter	Reduced-fat Greek yoghurt with defrosted frozen berries and seeds or nuts

WEEKLY MEAL PLANS

Conclusion

Here's one final hack: the advice in this book isn't about "going on a diet" or eating differently as a short-term reset or health kick. These hacks can become daily habits for good.

Take what works for you and don't try to change everything at once. That might mean you start with cooking from scratch more frequently, ditching the fad diet or perhaps taking up a new sport that makes you smile.

Whatever hack you pick first, do so without any pressure to be perfect. We eat for nourishment and enjoyment as well as simple fuel and if we don't find good nutrition enjoyable, we won't stick to it. Neither should nutrition be rigid. There are no set-in-stone rules – eating well is about overall patterns, not striving for some unattainable ideal every day.

So find the hacks that help you personally prioritize a more balanced diet. There is no one-size-fits-all approach – ultimately, good nutrition is about discovering your own way of healthy eating that you can continue to enjoy for life.

Further reading

Allergy UK
Information for anyone living with an allergy or looking for a possible diagnosis.
www.allergyuk.org

Association for Nutrition
A searchable register of every qualified nutritionist in the UK.
www.associationfornutrition.org

BEAT
Support for anyone suffering with disordered eating.
www.beateatingdisorders.org.uk

British Dietetic Association
Find a qualified dietitian near you in the UK.
www.bda.uk.com

Coeliac UK
A charity for all those who need to live without gluten.
www.coeliac.org.uk

The Eatwell Guide
The UK government's at-a-glance infographic guide to a balanced diet.
www.gov.uk/government/publications/the-eatwell-guide

The Eatwell Guide adapted for vegans
www.vegansociety.com/resources/downloads/vegan-eatwell-guide

WWF Carbon Footprint Calculator
A free and quick tool to work out your score, including on food.
www.footprint.wwf.org.uk

Have you enjoyed this book?
If so, why not write a review on your favourite website?

If you're interested in finding out more about our books, find us on Facebook at **Summersdale Publishers**, on Twitter/X at **@Summersdale** and on Instagram, TikTok and Bluesky at **@summersdalebooks** and get in touch.
We'd love to hear from you!

Thanks very much for buying this Summersdale book.
www.summersdale.com

Image credits

Cover and pp.1, 3, 7, 29, 33, 47, 64, 151 © DesignByS/Shutterstock.com; all photos by Emily Kerrigan; p.9 © Anastasiia Usenko/Shutterstock.com; p.11 © Anastasiia Usenko/Shutterstock.com; ivector/Shutterstock.com (crisps); GoodStudio/Shutterstock.com (doughnut); p.13 © Anastasiia Usenko/Shutterstock.com; p.15 © Anastasiia Usenko/Shutterstock.com (food icons); ngupakarti/Shutterstock.com (kale); p.17 © Anastasiia Usenko/Shutterstock.com; Rica Nohara/Shutterstock.com (tofu); p.19 © V.studio/Shutterstock.com (fork); Anastasiia Usenko/Shutterstock.com (food); p.21 © Anastasiia Usenko/Shutterstock.com; p.25 © elenabsl/Shutterstock.com; pp.26–7 © Anastasiia Usenko/Shutterstock.com; p.29 © V.studio/Shutterstock.com (fork); Anastasiia Usenko/Shutterstock.com (food); p.31 © Anastasiia Usenko/Shutterstock.com; p.33 © V.studio/Shutterstock.com (fork); DesignByS/Shutterstock.com (food); p.34 – The Eatwell Guide © of the Crown; p.35 © Anastasiia Usenko/Shutterstock.com (fizzy drinks); ivector/Shutterstock.com (crisps); mentalmind/Shutterstock.com (salt); p.36 © DesignByS/Shutterstock.com (single potato); ivector/Shutterstock.com (crisps and chips); instant mash by Summersdale Publishers; p.37 © V.studio/Shutterstock.com (fork); p.45 © HeyWorld/Shutterstock.com (Mediterranean bits); Look_Studio/Shutterstock.com (lobster dinner); KENJIROU MORITA/Shutterstock.com (ramen); p.51 © GoodStudio/Shutterstock.com (fish and cheese); DesignByS/Shutterstock.com (carrot and strawberry); Viktoriia Lapshyna/Shutterstock.com (bread); GoodStudio/Shutterstock.com (doughnut, pizza, can); mentalmind/Shutterstock.com (honey stick and salt); HeyWorld/Shutterstock.com (olive oil); p.55 © DesignByS/Shutterstock.com (whole and slice of apple); Brothers klia/Shutterstock.com (juice carton); p.57 © V.studio/Shutterstock.com (fork); Anastasiia Usenko/Shutterstock.com (food); p.59 © Adisak Riwkratok/Shutterstock.com; p.62 © ClassicVector/Shutterstock.com; pp.67 and 83 © Yuliia Konakhovska/Shutterstock.com (arrows); p.72 © MicroOne/Shutterstock.com (porridge); Zaikinles/Shutterstock.com (salad); Tetiana Maltseva/Shutterstock.com (pasta); p.74 © Ihor Biliavskyi/Shutterstock.com; p.76 © Oleksandr Drypsiak/Shutterstock.com (takeaway coffee cups); kichikimi/Shutterstock.com (soda can); asya_su/Shutterstock.com (teabag); Takoyaki Tech/Shutterstock.com (energy drink); p.77 © Blueastro/Shutterstock.com (wine bottle); Incomible/Shutterstock.com (wine glass, shot glass); Julia Anisimova/Shutterstock.com (beer bottle, beer glass); p.79 © Design.X_X/Shutterstock.com (red meat), WinWinFolly/Shutterstock.com (fish); GoodStudio/Shutterstock.com (eggs); Dyz11/Shutterstock.com (pulses); HappyPictures/Shutterstock.com (fish in packet); ivector/Shutterstock.com (canned food and frozen food tubs); lemono/Shutterstock.com (veg plate); Chernyka/Shutterstock.com (chilli); byherline/Shutterstock.com (herbs); GoodStudio/Shutterstock.com (paper food packets); Iconic Bestiary/Shutterstock.com (meals on trays); vectorstudi/Shutterstock.com (spaghetti); LadadikArt/Shutterstock.com (rice); p.84 © DesignByS/Shutterstock.com; p.85 © DesignByS/Shutterstock.com; pp.89 and 160 © V.studio/Shutterstock.com (fork)